A Twentieth Century Fund Book

The Twentieth Century Fund sponsors and supervises timely analyses of economic policy, foreign affairs, and domestic political issues. Not-for-profit and nonpartisan, the Fund was founded in 1919 and endowed by Edward A. Filene.

The Most Useful Gift

Jeffrey Prottas

Foreword by
Richard C. Leone

The Most Useful Gift

*Altruism and the Public Policy
of Organ Transplants*

A Twentieth Century Fund Book

Jossey-Bass Publishers • San Francisco

Substantial discounts on bulk quantities of Jossey-Bass books are available to corporations, professional associations, and other organizations. For details and discount information, contact the special sales department at Jossey-Bass Inc., Publishers. (415) 433-1740; Fax (415) 433-0499.

For sales outside the United States, contact Maxwell Macmillan International Publishing Group, 866 Third Avenue, New York, New York 10022.

Manufactured in the United States of America. Nearly all Jossey-Bass books, jackets, and periodicals are printed on recycled paper that contains at least 50 percent recycled waste, including 10 percent postconsumer waste. Many of our materials are also printed with vegetable-based ink; during the printing process these inks emit fewer volatile organic compounds (VOCs) than petroleum-based inks. VOCs contribute to the formation of smog.

Library of Congress Cataloging-in-Publication Data

Prottas, Jeffrey, date.
  The most useful gift / altruism and the public policy of organ transplants / Jeffrey Prottas : foreword by Richard C. Leone. — 1st ed.
    p. cm. — (The Jossey-Bass health series)
  Includes bibliographical references and index.
  ISBN 1-55542-644-1
  1. Donation of organs, tissues, etc.—Social aspects—United States. 2. Transplantation of organs, tissues, etc.—Social aspects—United States. 3. Donation of organs, tissues, etc.— Government policy—United States. 4. Transplantation of organs, tissues, etc.—Government policy—United States. 5. Donation of organs, tissues, etc.—United States—Moral and ethical aspects. 6. Transplantation of organs, tissues, etc.—United States—Moral and ethical aspects. I. Title. II. Series.
  [DNLM: 1. Altruism. 2. Organ Transplantation. 3. Public Policy— United States. 4. Organ Procurement. WO 660 P967a 1994]
  RD129.5.P76 1994
  362.1'783—dc20
  DNLM/DLC
  for Library of Congress   93-38239
                                                                      CIP

FIRST EDITION
HB Printing   10 9 8 7 6 5 4 3 2 1   Code 9436

The Jossey-Bass Health Series

Contents

List of Tables

Foreword

WE ARE UNDOUBTEDLY LIVING on the leading edge of a revolution not only in the technology of medicine and biology but also—inevitably—in the ethical and policy issues raised by current and imminent developments. The next few generations of humans will come to look at fundamental questions about life differently. In a sense, they will hold the very concept of life up to a bright new light, peering inside at the essence of their humanity. We have precious little experience to guide us. But in one area, at least, we are accumulating knowledge and experience about such complex, even troubling questions. For yesterday's miracle of transplanted organs has become, if not routine, at least a normal part of medicine.

Organ transplantation is different from other high-technology medical procedures. While many individual operations have provoked controversy, the transplant industry itself has received near-universal support and facilitation from federal and state governments and the blessing of most religions and cultures. It differs too in that while constant improvements have been made in the areas of immunosuppressive drugs and transplant techniques, these advances have not driven up the real costs of, or demand for, the procedure. The determining factor remains the human organ itself: each operation would be impossible without the generous gift made by an organ donor.

Unfortunately, due to a constant shortage of transplantable organs, this unique requirement results in the painful reality that, unlike other medical decisions involving life and death, the allocation of life to one patient at the cost of the life of others is a rare event outside of transplantation.

Perhaps because of the altruistic nature of organ donation, transplantation programs are often evaluated in ethical terms rather than just in technical and economic terms. More so than with other medical treatments, transplants are often above the usual considerations of health administration. Public policy and public attitudes have granted the industry special considerations: close to two-thirds of organ transplants are paid for directly by public funds, and government funding makes the organ procurement infrastructure possible. It seems that, in return, the industry is held to high ethical standards: federal law prohibits the purchasing of organs for transplant; those involved in patient care and those involved in organ procurement may not be the same people; organ distribution is decided according to a strict set of rules.

In his investigation into the technological, organizational, and ethical dimensions of organ transplantation, Jeffrey Prottas, research professor at Brandeis University and deputy director of the Institute for Health Policy at the Heller Graduate School, has provided us with a thoughtful and engaging discussion of the issues. Grounding his analysis in a long-term involvement at the intersection of organ transplantation and public policy, Prottas reveals the system's successes and failures and underscores the challenges that remain.

The Twentieth Century Fund has sponsored several projects examining the fate of the nation's health. *The Most Useful Gift* takes its place next to recent studies such as Malvin Schechter's *Beyond Medicare* (1993) and Bradford Gray's *The Profit Motive and Patient Care* (1991). Jeffrey Prottas brings a weath of knowledge to this project, and the Fund is grateful to him for undertaking this effort.

New York, New York
January 1994

Richard C. Leone
President
The Twentieth Century Fund

Preface

ORGAN TRANSPLANTATION is an extraordinary technical achievement. Success requires not only advanced surgical techniques but also the application of some of the most advanced pharmaceuticals in existence. These drugs—immunosuppressives—are used to undermine the human body's essential defensive immunological system to circumvent organ rejection. Their use requires treading the finest of lines between organ rejection and opportunistic infection. This is high-technology medicine at its most recondite.

But immunosuppressive drugs are of primitive simplicity compared to the organs they are used to protect. No technology compares in complexity and subtlety with the workings of a human liver or kidney. And these organs cannot be manufactured, grown, or purchased; they can be obtained only as gifts from the families of the dead.

This process, extending from acts of altruism in the midst of tragedy to high-technology medicine, is the subject of *The Most Useful Gift*.

Background

More than two decades ago, a British social theorist named Richard Titmus wrote a book about blood donation, *The Gift Relationship*. In it he examined the operational and ethical implications of obtaining a critical medical supply—human blood—by donation. He concluded that both the quality of the blood and the quality of society were enhanced by treating blood as a gift rather than a commodity. Coincidentally, within a year of the publication of his book, the United States Congress began a program that initiated the development of a nationwide system for procuring and transplanting human organs obtained as gifts.

Organs differ from blood in a great many ways. They cannot be renewed; one cannot both give and keep an organ. Humans have two kidneys, but no other organs can be given while a person is alive. This fact changes both the locus of giving to the family and the circumstance of giving to a sudden death. But a public system dedicated to obtaining organs as gifts raises many of the same questions raised by Titmus: How does a society organize the "harvesting" and "distribution" of such gifts? What are the roles of families, doctors, and public bodies in such a system? What obligations are incurred when a lifesaving medical system is constructed on a foundation of acts of altruism?

These questions become more salient in a time when the rationing of medical care is a major item on the national agenda. Organ transplantation as high-technology medicine can be treated much as other expensive medical technologies are treated—both Oregon and New Jersey consider organ transplantation in this light. In this context, rationing issues naturally arise. Yet organs differ from other medical commodities in that they are obtained via a public system without payment and as an act of kindness. On that basis, perhaps, they ought to be treated differently.

In this sense, organ transplantation and the public infra-structure that makes it possible raise questions about the role of public policy in bridging social, medical, and economic issues and defining the lines between them. This is an issue of potential importance to policy makers. It is increasingly clear that in this area, issues of economic policy, health care policy, and social equity merge in ways previously unconsidered. Organ transplantation highlights many of those issues particularly starkly.

Ethical issues in public policy are similarly highlighted by the conundrums of organ transplantation policy. How can the efficient use of organs be reconciled with their fair distribution? How can the concerns of medical professionals and their duties to their patients be reconciled with the broader responsibilities of a public system to both donor families and patients awaiting organs?

Finally, there are operational issues. The organ procurement system is an organizational innovation in response to technological change. In a world where there is a general sense that human institutions fail to control or adapt to change, analysis of the successes, failures, and conflicts in the organ procurement system are of interest to social observers and to managers facing analogous challenges.

My involvement in this system started with studies of the effectiveness of organ procurement organizations. My work slowly expanded in focus from questions of organizational effectiveness to an examination of the motivations of those involved in the donation process and the ways decisions regarding organ use are made. Finally I became directly involved in organ transplantation policy with my appointment to the National

Task Force on Organ Transplantation. *The Most Useful Gift* brings together in one place what I have learned and come to believe about organ transplantation over almost twenty years.

Overview of the Contents

This book is divided into six chapters. Chapter One sets the stage for consideration of organ transplantation as modern high-technology medicine capable of saving the desperately ill—but at great financial cost. Organ transplantation leaves its beneficiaries dependent on continued medical care for the rest of their lives. I also examine the role that public action has played in the development of organ transplantation. Because organs must be obtained as gifts from newly dead cadavers, an extensive legal and organizational infrastructure is necessary if transplantation is to be done on a large scale. In the United States, this infrastructure has grown rapidly.

Chapter Two describes in detail the nation's system for procuring transplantable organs. This system is a large-scale organizational innovation developed for the sole purpose of maintaining the supply of these organs. Over time, the system has changed toward increased public involvement and oversight. Concerns about the supply of organs and about their fair use have led to a very high level of government oversight of the organ procurement system.

Chapter Three deals with the public's role. The willingness of Americans to support organ donation defines the supply of organs available for transplantation. Social and economic factors influence that willingness. More proximately, the attitudes of the families of potential donors determine how many people with end-stage organ failure can be saved.

Chapter Four considers the attitudes and role of the medical personnel involved. Medical professionals—doctors and nurses in intensive care units primarily—also play a key role in determining the success of organ procurement efforts. They are central to the procurement process. Only they can identify potential donors in time and only they can declare brain death. Medical professionals are in principle willing to perform tasks related to organ procurement but in practice find some of them difficult or threatening.

Chapter Five shifts attention from the procurement of organs to their distribution. Organs are in chronically short supply, and their distribution is a zero-sum game. About one-third of patients awaiting a heart transplant die before they can receive a graft. This chapter traces the issues of organ allocation and discusses the institutions and the politics involved in resolving those issues.

Finally, Chapter Six is about the public policy implications of organ transplantation and the nature of the obligations incurred. I argue that transplantation is unique and that special public policy obligations arise from that uniqueness. Of course, transplantation is high-technology medicine and shares many important characteristics with this category. However, it is also qualitatively different from other medical technologies in that human organs cannot be manufactured, can be obtained only as gifts, and are sacred objects from a psychological and cultural point of view. The book ends with an argument for the public funding of all organ transplants to ensure equal access to all Americans.

The Most Useful Gift tells an encouraging story. In contrast to our experiences with reproductive technologies and technologies that prolong the lives of the dying, we have responded quickly and, by and large, effectively to organ transplantation. We have constructed new institutions, altered our expectations of established ones, mobilized public opinion, and developed new legal and ethical systems appropriate to our newly expanded technical capacities. This book considers the changes we have brought about, evaluates our institutions and methods, and discusses the public policy implications and challenges that remain.

Acknowledgments

There are some four hundred transplant coordinators working in the United States. Scores of them have educated me and helped me understand the system that they make possible, and many have become my friends. But the acknowledgment they deserve is not really for their contribution to this book but rather for their contribution to organ transplantation and to the lives saved and enhanced by it. Often underpaid, generally underappreciated, always overworked, they serve organ donor families and organ transplant recipients equally. Without their routinely extraordinary efforts, neither this book nor organ transplantation would be possible.

Without the support and collaboration of my colleagues at Brandeis University, especially Helen Batten, the research on which this book is based could not have been done. Without the support of the Twentieth Century Fund, it would have been impossible to use this research to inform the larger policy and ethical issues of organ transplantation.

Waltham, Massachusetts   Jeffrey Prottas
January 1994

The Author

JEFFREY PROTTAS is research professor at Brandeis University and deputy director of the Institute for Health Policy at the Heller Graduate School there. He received his B.A. degree (1969) from Colgate University and his Ph.D. degree (1975) in political science from the Massachusetts Institute of Technology.

Prottas's main areas of research have been the impact of technological change on organizations and the implementation of public policy. He has directed research on hospital emergency rooms, long-term care facilities, Medicaid managed-care organizations, housing authorities, and organ procurement organizations. He is currently involved in studies of state drug diversion control programs, the role of county government in health care delivery, and a national evaluation of the nation's tissue-banking system.

Prottas has chaired the organ procurement subcommittee of the National Task Force on Organ Transplantation, has served on the State of Massachusetts Organ Donation and Transplant Advisory Committee, and is a trustee of the New England Organ bank and a member of the Core Clinical Advisory Group to the Commissioner of Health of New Jersey. He is the author of *People-Processing: The Street-Level Bureaucrat in Public Bureaucracies* (1979) as well as more than a score of articles on organ donation and transplantation.

The Most
Useful Gift

1

Foundations
of Transplantation

ORGAN TRANSPLANTATION in the United States de-
pends on several factors all coming together. These factors include the development of medical technologies, especially immunosuppressive drugs to inhibit the rejection of the transplant;
government support in terms of financing and laws; a nationwide infrastructure capable of locating donors; and a population willing to act generously by permitting donation. What
is unique about this list is its breadth. At one extreme, it contains the development of highly advanced biotechnology; at the
other, a widespread public altruism; and in between, public policies designed to allow technology and kindness to support one
another.

In this chapter, we will survey the transplantation system
and its foundations. In the chapters that follow, we will address
the ethical and policy implications of its unique co-dependence
on the most advanced of technologies and the most basic of
human experiences.

A Successful Technology

The transplantation of a human organ from one person to
another is magic. For centuries, perhaps millennia, such an undertaking has been a dream. Total ignorance of both infection
control and human immunology made it virtually impossible for

the dream to come true until the second half of the twentieth century.

It was not until 1954 that the first even marginally successful kidney transplant was performed in the United States, at the Massachusetts General Hospital. The donor and recipient were identical twins. Since then, medical technology has apparently "routinized" magic of various sorts. In 1991, more than sixteen thousand human organ transplants were done in the United States alone (United Network for Organ Sharing, 1992). This is magic on a grand scale: it has become an industry.

In 1992, more than eight hundred organ transplantation programs were operating in the United States, including kidney programs, heart programs, liver programs, heart-lung programs, and still experimental pancreas programs. Advances in surgical techniques and drug therapies have made it possible—with varying degrees of success—to transplant most of the major vascularized organs. In 1992, almost 10,000 kidneys were transplanted, 2,100 hearts, 3,000 livers, 500 pancreases, and 450 other vascularized organs, mostly lungs (United Network for Organ Sharing, 1992). The total cost of this industry is not negligible, either to the federal government, which pays for virtually all kidney transplants, or for private insurance, HMOs, Medicaid, and other insurers, which in various combinations pay for most others. Best estimates are that these procedures cost about $200 million in 1990.

Organ transplantation is a thriving medical industry because the procedure actually works—not always and not for always, but in most cases and often for a long time. The survival rate of a heart transplant after one year is over 80 percent. The figure is similar for liver and kidney transplants.

Over time, the function of a transplant declines. Whereas 80 percent of transplanted organs are viable at the end of one year, by the end of five years that percentage has dropped—to 60 percent for kidneys, for example, although some patients continue to do well after ten years and longer, and even those whose kidney is rejected after five years are perfectly capable of receiving another with every probability of another long period of success. The long-term viability of nonrenal transplants is less clear. Complications still endanger transplanted hearts after about five years, and both heart and liver transplants are too new as widely employed technologies to permit generalization about their long-term viability. Unlike renal transplantation patients, however, heart and liver recipients face imminent death in the absence of a transplant. For a patient with six months to live, five years of reasonably healthy life with a new heart is an attractive alternative. Despite the need for lifelong immunosuppressive therapy, most transplant patients are functional and capable of living fairly normal lives.

Strict selection criteria are imposed on transplant recipients. Only patients with total organ system failure are considered suitable candidates. Heart and liver recipients especially must be carefully screened, and a difficult balance is sought. On the one hand, only clearly and imminently terminal patients are appropriate. On the other hand, transplantable organs are in very short supply, and so they must be used for patients who have a high probability of not rejecting them. This is reflected in the selection criteria, which favor younger recipients with no other underlying illness, early in the course of their disease, before its debilitating effects have diminished their resilience. The selection of optimal transplant patients therefore involves objective criteria and subjective clinical judgment—all in a context in which people in need will die. Although many medical decisions involve life and death, the stark allocation of life to one patient at the cost of the life of others is rare outside of transplantation.

Transplantation is not limited to organs: many types of human tissue are transplanted from one person to another. In fact, the use of tissue in medical procedures is far more common than the use of human organs, primarily because tissue is far more plentiful. There are about one hundred eye banks in the United States, and in 1992 they procured approximately ninety-two thousand corneas from some forty-five thousand donors. That is more than ten times the number of donors in the organ procurement system. About forty-two thousand corneal implants were done in 1992, more than three times the number of organ transplants. However, the American eye-banking system is organizationally, legally, and medically distinct from the organ procurement and transplantation system and so will not be systematically discussed in this book (Eye Bank Association, 1992).

The same is true of the nation's skin-banking system. Skin banks operate separately and differently from the organ procurement system. Although the same laws apply to skin banking as to organ procurement, that is the extent of the overlap between them.

Human bone, tendons, fascia, and similar tissue are also transplanted. Data on musculoskeletal tissue banking (generally referred to as bone banking because bone is its central product) are scanty. The number of bone donors in 1992 was estimated at between 4,000 and 6,500—a scale comparable to organ procurement. Indeed, between one-third and one-half of all organ donors are also tissue donors. However, because human bone is generally used in the form of small vials of bone powder or chips, the "units" of bone used in medical procedures number in the hundreds of thousands. Traditionally, bone banking has been separate from organ procurement, but in recent years, some organizations have begun to engage in both. The two activities share the same basic legal foundation and depend on many of the same medical professionals and families. The ethical issues are likewise similar, and most of what will be said in these pages about organ procurement and public attitudes also apply to tissue procurement. These overlaps mean that the relationship between organ and musculoskeletal tissue procurement is becoming a serious policy concern. However, the issue remains one of interorganizational relationships because the organ and tissue procurement systems are distinct and face different problems. Throughout this book, reference will be made to tissue procurement issues when organ procurement issues touch on them. However, no systematic examination of tissue procurement or transplantation is contained here. Tissue banking is too large and complex an issue to be treated in passing in a book on organ transplantation.

Xenografts will not be systematically discussed. Every few months, newspapers report some startling new experiment in the transplantation of an animal organ into a human. Such xenografts are experiments and have little or no direct relationship to the organ procurement and transplantation system or with the public policies supporting it; only the surgeons involved are the same. In general, the recipients of these animal organs are not candidates for human organ transplants. Given the universal failure of xenografts, it would be inappropriate to perform one on a patient who might otherwise receive a human organ. Xenografts are in such an early stage of development and their future is so uncertain that they remain largely irrelevant to transplantation practice and policy. Xenografts may ultimately represent a partial solution to the chronic shortage of transplantable human organs, but not even the most sanguine observers expect this to occur in the immediate future.

A Very Modern Technology

Even though organ transplantation is a medical activity of surpassing complexity, recent technical advances have not, as they generally do in medical care, driven up the real cost of the procedure. A transplanted organ is foreign tissue, and the body's immune system treats it as a dangerous invader. The natural result is acute rejection—the rapid and comprehensive destruction of the new organ. Successful transplantation is therefore built on the development of substances that suppress this immunological response. These immunosuppressive drugs are among the most advanced biotechnical agents in existence, but their use requires training, experience, and continual midcourse corrections. Even the most widely used of these new drugs, cyclosporine, is a blunt instrument in comparison to the wondrous complexity and subtlety of the human immunological system. The greatest advantage of cyclosporine is that it is a more focused agent than those previously employed and does not weaken all aspects of the body's immunological defenses. However, it does not act so specifically as to prevent rejection of the transplanted organ without compromising the patient's resistance to other invasions, such as infections. The use of this drug therefore requires treading a narrow and shifting path between organ rejection and serious infectious illness.

Organ recipients must take immunosuppressive drugs for the rest of their lives to maintain this delicate balance. In this respect, organ transplantation is typical of high-technology medicine in the late twentieth century: it saves lives but increases chronic illness.

Organ transplantation is the social paradox of modern medicine in distilled form. It is a very expensive procedure. Yet transplants are, to varying degrees, both cost-effective and medically efficacious. The existence of dialysis makes kidney transplantation actually economical. And the high success rates of heart and liver transplantation both give good cost-per-year-of-life-saved ratios, superior to a great many routine treatments administered for certain cancers, for example. In addition, they permit a reasonable quality of life.

At the same time, curing organ failure through transplantation comes at the price of permanent dependence on powerful and very dangerous drugs that expose a person to increased illness risk from infection. They are also expensive. The older, less effective immunosuppressives cost around $800 a year; the newest ones, about $7,000. So, as with many chronic illnesses, treatment success in transplantation depends on the merging of highly sophisticated biotechnical agents and social and financial support systems. Careful lifelong drug compliance is a precondition for long-term graft survival. Good insurance coverage and good earning ability are also very helpful.

Finally, although success in organ transplantation depends on advanced medical tools and skills, the most complex, sophisticated, and powerful piece in the process—the human organ itself—is not manufactured but grown. And it is obtained by the decision of a family dealing with the sudden death of one of its members. If organ transplantation is a twenty-first-century activity, death and grieving are as old as humankind and probably not much changed since the beginning.

Organ Donation

For all our extraordinary advances in medicine, we have yet to produce a fully adequate substitute for any human organ. Functionally, the heart is the simplest organ that we have tried to replicate. In fact, heart-lung machines that support life during surgery and in other short-term emergency circumstances are in common use. However, these are unsuitable for longer use because of their size, power requirements, and need for professional monitoring. Artificial hearts have been implanted in several patients but so unsuccessfully that the program has been halted. Present technology has no substitution, no matter how short term or inadequate, for the human liver. Artificial kidney machines are a partial success: although they can filter blood well enough to maintain life, they cannot perform the little-understood endocrine functions of the kidney.

Treatment for end-stage organ failure—the only treatment in the case of heart and liver failure and the best treatment in the case of renal failure—therefore depends on human organs, obtained via voluntary donation.

The organs we are considering are not renewable. Unlike blood and bone marrow, which can be both donated and kept, hearts, livers, kidneys, lungs, and pancreas will not grow again. Organs can be donated only when the donor no longer has any use for them—that is, when the donor is dead.

As in so many other ways, kidneys are a limited exception to this rule. People have two kidneys, and one is quite adequate for a normal life. It is possible to obtain a kidney from a living donor with minimal risk to the donor, and in the United States some two thousand kidneys a year (25 percent of the total) are obtained in this way ("HCFA Releases 1991 . . . ," 1993). In general, only the family of a recipient is approached.

In Europe, virtually no living related donors are used, in part because the European medical community does not consider the practice of removing a functioning organ ethically acceptable and in part thanks to the excellent results of cadaveric transplantation.

Public Support

Even in the United States, most kidneys and, of course, all other organs come from cadaveric donors. Organ transplantation starts with death, usually a tragic one, since most organs come from people in their twenties who until their death were in good health and free of systemic disease. Furthermore, organs deteriorate very rapidly after their blood supply has been cut off. This means that acceptable donors must die in a hospital and be declared brain-dead—a determination made when there is total and permanent cessation of all brain activity, including that in the brain stem. Under such circumstances, the cadaver's heart can be kept beating artificially and the organs protected until removed and cooled. Consequently, central nervous system trauma is the typical cause of death among organ donors, usually caused by automobile or other accidents (40–50 percent); homicides and strokes are also common causes of death for organ donors (Prottas and Batten, 1991a). Thus organ donation is possible only as a result of nightmarish tragedy. The archetypical situation is the sudden accidental death of a healthy son. More often than not, a mother will have to decide to allow her son's body to be dismembered within twenty-four hours; when asked, about 70 percent of families agree (Prottas and Batten, 1991b).

Public support for organ donation is not a worldwide phenomenon. Many cultures with the technical means of doing organ transplantation are unable to operate a significant program because they lack public support. For example, Japan has mastered the medical techniques, but Japanese culture provides little or no support for the procedures. In contrast, Western culture is highly supportive, including all major American religions. The Catholic church officially encourages donation, as evidenced by a papal proclamation. Protestant denominations that have expressed a position are strongly supportive. Among Jews, only the ultraorthodox object to organ donation. Although Jewish law forbids the mutilation of cadavers, even Conservative rabbis have argued that because saving a life supersedes any such prohibition, organ donation is justified. The complex logic that extends this reasoning to nonlifesaving donations such as corneas is instructive as an instance of Talmudic thought and of the profound commitment of Western culture to placing the needs of the living over the rights of the dead (United Network for Organ Sharing, 1991a). There is a widely shared consensus that organ donation has a strong positive moral value.

There is also a consensus that decisions regarding donation ought to be made by the deceased's family. As we shall see, by law, the donation decision can be made by the donor in a premortem statement. However, American practice is to defer to the wishes of the deceased's family. Organ donations are social decisions and respond to cultural realities far weightier than the acts of state legislatures.

Families decide to make organ donations as part of the process of coming to terms with the death of a loved one. The universality of respect for the family's role is such that even in nations where the law does not require family consent, it is generally requested. Doctors, nurses, and organ procurement coordinators all partake of the culture that gives families a right to resolve such intimate issues themselves.

What is less evident is the social character and importance of organ donation. The decision to permit a donation is a decision to help a stranger. For this reason, it helps define a community and moral behavior within that community. It is a sacred act that can make death more meaningful, less useless, more bearable. In this way, an act that is essentially private takes on social and moral importance. This complex nature makes organ donation unique as the foundation of a high-technology form of health care. It also makes it subject to public action on both the symbolic and practical levels.

Legal Foundation

American law has been exceptionally supportive of organ donation and transplantation. The financial and organizational foundation of transplantation in the United States is the End-Stage Renal Disease (ESRD) program. Passed by Congress as an amendment to the Medicare program, the ESRD program includes all persons covered by Social Security who suffer from renal failure and need dialysis or a kidney transplant. It classifies these individuals as disabled and thereby makes them eligible for Medicare coverage.

Public expense for transplantation is substantial, and the payment system for organ procurement is unique. Before 1983, Medicare reimbursed hospitals 80 percent of actual medical

costs. But under the ESRD program, 100 percent of organ procurement costs would be paid. These new rules fostered the development of a nationwide organ procurement system. At one
time, almost a hundred organizations were being wholly funded
by the ESRD program. In 1983—when the Medicare system
abandoned cost-based reimbursement in favor of prospective
payment—a kidney transplantation payment rate was developed,
but the cost-based, 100 percent reimbursement practice was
maintained for procurement. Organ procurement has always
had a unique place in federal health care policy.

In effect, the ESRD program mandates national health insurance for a specific illness category. Transplantation was singled
out again in 1986 when Congress required that immunosuppressive drugs be paid for with public funds—making them the
only outpatient drugs covered by Medicare.

While the federal government has provided the financial
foundation for transplantation, state governments have provided
the legal foundation. Every state has passed the Uniform Anatomical Gift Act (UAGA), formulated in the late 1960s by the
national Conference of Commissioners on Uniform State Laws
(Intergovernmental Health Policy Project, 1985). The UAGA
sets the basic legal ground rules for organ procurement in the
United States, recognizes the right of an individual and the immediate family to donate organs, and specifies who has the right
to make such a donation. The deceased individual has the first
and deciding voice, which can be exercised by means of an organ donation card, which is, under UAGA, a legally binding
document. To facilitate their signing, many states have made
such cards part of the driver's license (another indication of the
level of official support for organ donation). If the deceased has

not expressed a preference, the UAGA specifies a priority order in which relatives have the right to make a donation decision, usually spouse, then parents, then less direct kin, and ultimately the medical examiner or similar official if no relative can be found. This means that organs may legally be removed if no responsible relative can be located. It also means that a signed donor card legally supersedes the wishes of spouse or mother.

This aspect of the law is sufficiently out of step with social practices, however, for it never to be employed. In practice, the family is always asked, and a signed card is never used to override the family's preference. The cultural belief that this sort of decision is a familial one is so strong that even in nations such as France, Spain, and Austria where the law allows organ retrieval without family permission, the family is routinely asked.

The UAGA rules regarding who may donate provides legal support to the giving side of the "gift of life." Its provisions regarding who may receive are also supportive of organ donation. The law provides exceptional protection for medical personnel against lawsuits involving organ donation so long as these professionals acted "in good faith." This is probably the broadest protection granted any medical procedure. In fact, there has never been a successful suit arising from an organ donation in the United States.

The final part of the law requires that the people involved in the patient's care and those involved in organ procurement not be the same people. In particular, determination of death must not be made by a physician with an interest in organ retrieval. The normal division of labor in medicine ensures this practice in any case—neurophysicians are usually involved in brain death determinations, transplant surgeons in organ procurement. The latter lack the expertise to make the death determination, and the former have no occasion to transplant organs. Nevertheless, this aspect of the law precludes any suggestion of a conflict of interest.

The prerequisite for organ donation is a declaration of brain death, which is an uncontroversial concept among physicians. Nevertheless, they have welcomed state involvement in this area, and laws have been enacted that specifically recognize the determination of death by brain death criteria. States' willingness to enter into such a technical medical area reflects their desire to reassure physicians of the legitimacy of the organ procurement process.

Given the UAGA's emphasis on the explicit and voluntary nature of organ donation, the anomaly of medical examiner laws is worthy of note. These laws do not apply to vascularized organs but in effect mandate a "presumed consent" practice for certain human tissues—primarily corneas and, in some cases, pituitary glands. ("Presumed consent" means that the law presumes that consent would be given if asked for and so allows the procurement to go forth unless the family spontaneously expresses disapproval.) What is striking about medical examiner laws in the United States is that they are quite out of step with the ethos of the organ donation system. In fact, the presumed consent approach is universally rejected for organ donation and has failed in other countries, yet as applied here to corneas, it has engendered virtually no public outcry.

In 1986, the federal government (and a majority of state legislatures) again entered the organ donation field with legislation imposing, as a condition of Medicare reimbursement, a system of "required request/routine inquiry." Routine inquiry laws require that the family of every medically suitable potential donor be given the option of permitting organ and tissue donation. In the federal law and most state laws, this obligation is imposed on the hospital, making it mandatory for every hospital to have procedures to approach every potential donor family (Caplan and Welvang, 1989).

Unfortunately, these laws have not had much impact on the supply of organs, but they do represent an important extension of government involvement in medical practice. They deny the physician the right to make judgments about the suitability of organ donors beyond the purely technical ones; referral of clinically appropriate donors to the "procurement people" is now mandatory. As virtually any person dying in a hospital is suitable as a tissue donor, in principle the hospital must have a system whereby virtually every family is asked if they wish to allow organ or tissue removal.

In practice, the impact of routine inquiry laws is slight, but the message is clear that the medical profession has an obligation to cooperate in organ procurement. These laws have laid out a second, equally important public principle—that society's commitment to transplantation is sufficiently important to justify governmental involvement in medical discretion. The level of public consensus on this is illustrated by the fact that these laws faced no resistance from medical associations and only minimal resistance from hospital groups, based not on an objection to the legitimacy of this approach but on a desire to avoid additional paperwork!

The UAGA and brain death laws are state-level statutes that provide the legal sanction for organ donation. The federal role, originally limited to provide the financial support for the program, has expanded to include moral considerations. In early 1983, stories began to emerge about proposals to purchase kidneys for transplantation. Such actions were considered unethical by most of the transplantation community and were against the policy of all transplantation and procurement centers. However, it was not clear that there were legal prohibitions against paying donors for organs. Congress was sufficiently concerned to bring about a provision of the National Organ Transplantation Act specifically forbidding payment for organ donation. Though it is doubtful that this act has had much practical impact because the idea of paying for organs is so widely condemned, the American law against commercialization is symbolic. It places the federal government clearly behind a procurement system based on volunteerism and altruism and built around nonprofit organizations rather than for-profit firms.

The Organ Procurement Infrastructure

The organ procurement system was designed to "implement kindness," and the relationship between the family of a donor and the recipient can be called a "gift relationship" between strangers.

Organ procurement organizations (OPOs) are nonprofit organizations, either independently incorporated or associated with a hospital. At present, there are about seventy of them spread across the nation, each certified by the federal government. They are tied together by the national Organ Procurement and Transplantation Network (OPTN), a federally funded organization made up of transplant hospitals, organ procurement agencies, and public members with broad powers over organ sharing and procurement. While government involvement is extensive, operationally the origins of the organ procurement system are local and rooted in the medical care system.

Most OPOs were started by transplant surgeons facing a chronic insufficiency of organs. Fostering and directing an organization designed to locate suitable donors was an obvious step toward ensuring an adequate supply. As a result, organ procurement in the United States has always had a very solid base in the medical establishment at the local level. Its translocal infrastructure has generally been weaker, but not non-existent. There have been regional organizations fostering cooperation among centers, and, most important, there has been a national information system. This system, the United Network for Organ Sharing (UNOS), provided a computer listing of those awaiting a kidney transplant. While all aspects of the system are directly or indirectly federally funded, traditionally there has been only minimal federal oversight.

Organ procurement agencies are organizational adaptations to technological innovation. Most aspects of their operations are universal, responsive to the biological characteristics of human organs and the technical needs of transplantation (tissue typing and matching and organ preservation). The procedures are essentially the same around the world; donor identification, obtaining permission from families, and the distribution of organs, all of which have social aspects, might vary, but the cultural similarities of the Western world make even these processes surprisingly similar. Organ distribution is the most politicized step in the process and is subject to the greatest variation on the least substantial grounds.

The system is activated when an organ procurement organization—whose sole purpose is to locate, retrieve, and distribute transplantable organs—is informed by a hospital that a potential donor is dead or dying. After medical suitability is determined, representatives of the agency or the hospital will ask the patient's family to permit organ donation. If the answer is yes, the patient is maintained on a respirator (after death has been declared) to maintain a flow of blood to the organs, which are then removed in an operating room and immediately cooled to preserve them. The destination of the heart and liver will have been determined prior to removal, and these organs will be transported immediately to the hospital where the recipient is waiting in an operating room. The placement of kidneys must await the results of tissue typing and then tissue matching between donor and recipient; the distribution of kidneys, unlike that of hearts and livers, depends partly on histocompatibility. Most kidneys are transplanted in the locality in which they are procured, but the UNOS system allows appropriate patients to be identified in other parts of the country.

Public awareness of transplants and the symbolic issues arising from the use of human organs have greatly increased government involvement. Originally, government concern focused on the equity of organ distribution, based on the proposition that organs were not the property of the physician procuring them but of the public at large. The government also sought to improve the effectiveness of the procurement system and hence the total supply of organs. The result is that organ procurement and distribution are among the most carefully scrutinized aspects of the medical system.

All of the nation's OPOs are certified by the government, and the service area of each is government-defined. Each receives about two-thirds of its reimbursement from the ESRD program (the remainder comes from insurance companies paying for non-renal organs), and each must submit a comprehensive financial statement to the government. The translocal part of the organ procurement system operates directly under government contract.

The OPTN is federally funded, and membership is, in effect, mandatory for anyone involved in any aspect of organ transplantation. No nonmember organization may procure an organ, and no nonmember hospital may transplant one. The OPTN is made up primarily of organizations directly involved in transplantation and is in that sense almost a trade association. At the same time, it is closely tied to the government. Governmental bodies have required hospitals to cooperate with OPOs or risk losing their Medicare certification, have virtually eliminated competition among OPOs in the interests of effectiveness, and have dictated the makeup of the leadership of the organ procurement system at the national and local levels through legislation, all in the interest of equity. Indeed, so extensive is its governmental character that people both inside and outside the government argue that the OPTN is in effect a government agency and ought to be structured like one. In fact, the Department of Health and Human Services now insists on approving all OPTN policies. Beyond having provided financial support and a legal framework, public bodies have defined, organized, and controlled the way the organ procurement system operates. Organ procurement in the United States is public business.

2

The Organ
Procurement System

THE NATION'S organ procurement system consists of about seventy organ procurement organizations (OPOs). These agencies have the dual task of locating and procuring organs and then providing them to surgeons for transplantation. More abstractly, the system's task is to solicit the "gift of life" and then to make that gift meaningful by ensuring its use. Organizationally, this is a complex undertaking; it becomes even more so when considered as a moral enterprise. There are ethical obligations to donors as well as recipients, and both aspects are intensified and underscored by the public nature of the organ procurement system.

Understanding the nature of the organ procurement system is a precondition for understanding organ transplantation and transplantation policy in the United States. The first part of this chapter describes how OPOs operate to locate organ donors and to obtain usable human organs for transplantation. This is the publicly supported infrastructure of the transplantation industry.

It is worthy of study simply as an organizational response to technological innovation. Advances in immunosuppressive therapy and surgical techniques by themselves might result in several hundred organ transplants being done each year in the United States. The development of a nationwide system of agencies dedicated to locating organ donors makes fourteen thousand transplants possible.

Beyond this, the organ procurement system is also a vehicle for "exploiting" kindness. Public policy, solidly grounded in public attitudes, has decreed that organs may be obtained only as gifts. The organ procurement system is therefore structured to respond both to the technical needs of transplant teams and to the social and psychological needs of potential organ donors and their families. The concrete operational implications of this will be discussed. There are also ethical implications, some of which are reflected in how organs are procured and many of which must be confronted in how they are distributed.

Because donations must be obtained by appeals to altruism in particular and to moral values in general, the organ procurement system differs from other medical infrastructures. Its activities are legitimately evaluated not only in technical and economic terms but also in ethical terms. In the minds of the public—and of its members—the organ procurement system incurs a debt to organ donors to match their altruism with behavior on an analogous moral plain. In this sense, organ procurement is a moral enterprise, and standards of justice and kindliness not routinely applied to other institutions are applied to it. The fact that the organ procurement system is also a public system funded by public money and buttressed by law increases its uniqueness.

Public Involvement

The organ procurement system resulted from congressional passage of the End-Stage Renal Disease (ESRD) Act of 1972. In the late 1960s and early 1970s, medical progress made it possible to prolong indefinitely the life of a person without functioning kidneys through hemodialysis (the artificial filtration of blood to remove waste products). However, the procedure was prohibitively expensive, making rationing necessary. "God committees" determined who would live—who would have access to the lifesaving dialysis machines—and who would die.

This was not a stable situation, certainly not in the affluent early 1970s, and pressure for the government to accept financial responsibility became strong. The medical profession supported government involvement, and Congress was assured that the size of the dependent population would not be excessive. In 1967, the prestigious Gottschalk Report estimated that only four or five thousand new dialysis patients would appear each year (Fox and Swazey, 1973), and as late as 1972, estimates of only 7,500 new patients were widely accepted. Yet in 1981, more than twenty-one thousand patients started dialysis for the first time, and by 1991, over 130,000 patients were being dialyzed at government expense.

Under the ESRD Act, renal failure was to be considered a disability entitling its victims to full coverage under the Medicare program. Although 90 percent of ESRD costs (and an even larger percentage of the attention of policy makers) were devoted to dialysis, Congress in fact expressed a general preference for transplantation as a means of dealing with renal failure. In part this reflected the medical view that a successful transplant was clinically superior to dialysis—although in 1972 only 50 percent were successful one year after surgery. In part it reflected Congress's belief that a transplant was a less costly solution. The ESRD Act therefore provided for 100 percent of organ procurement costs to be paid for by the federal government. In effect, this meant that the OPOs were fiscal drops for the ESRD program, under which all costs were paid by Medicare. Until the mid 1980s, when the procurement of nonrenal organs became a significant part of the work, the nation's OPOs received all of their funding from ESRD, even though they were never answerable to or under the direction of any government agency.

Government financing and improved clinical outcomes led to substantial growth in the size of the organ procurement system. In 1972, there were eight formally operational OPOs in the nation; ten years later, there were ten times that number. This growth reflected the assured financing of organ procurement and often the competition among transplant hospitals, each seeking to ensure a supply of organs for its transplant services. The growth in the number of OPOs continued until 1988, when federal regulations began to require that OPOs not compete within a single metropolitan area. Since then, the number of OPOs has actually been decreasing. The number is now around sixty-five.

Even in 1982, few areas of the nation were not served by some OPO, and today, no region is without such service. One inevitable result is that the average OPO is larger now than it was in the early 1980s.

The federal government has also influenced the structure of individual OPOs. Federal laws have altered the makeup of OPO boards of directors by requiring more public involvement (this subject will be discussed later). The indirect impact of federal policies has had at least as great an effect. Federal funding has underpinned the growth of the organ procurement system at the same time that policies have encouraged the merging of small OPOs into larger ones. The result has been that the average OPO serves more hospitals than in the early 1980s and has a larger and more professional staff. In 1982, two-thirds of OPOs were merely units of a hospital; now three-fourths are independently incorporated. In 1982, a full-time executive director was a rarity among OPOs; today, a large majority of OPOs employ one. Public action has thus contributed to the professionalization and growth of the individual OPOs that make up the organ procurement system (Prottas, 1985, 1989).

The Procurement Process

Every OPO must complete the same series of tasks to procure human organs. This is true regardless of the size of the OPO or its location. Indeed, the organ procurement process is essentially the same in all nations presently operating a large-scale system. Despite certain differences in law, the organ procurement process in the United States, Canada, and Western Europe faces the same challenges and follows the same rigid sequence of actions. Failure at any point means failure of the entire process. Some of these actions are wholly within the control of the OPO: maintenance of a donor, removal of organs, tissue typing, and organ placement. Others require the cooperation of outsiders. These latter actions are most problematical because cooperation from medical professionals and from the families of donors can only be requested, not required.

Referrals

The first step in the organ procurement process is the most important and the most difficult. Suitable organ donors appear at unpredictable times and under unforeseeable conditions. Automobile accidents, other traumas, and strokes are random events that do not inevitably lead to death, much less to death under conditions suitable for organ retrieval. Only the medical staff of the hospital treating a potential donor knows when all the prerequisites have come together.

When a hospital informs an OPO that a potential donor exists, this is called a referral. It is the most important step in the procurement process because without it, no process exists. Research has shown that failure to refer donors is the single greatest drag on organ supply.

Potential organ donors are reasonably easy for medical professionals in intensive care units (ICUs) to identify. They tend to be accident victims with trauma to the central nervous system—although stroke accounts for a significant secondary source of donors. The basic impediment to referral is social, not medical. Many referrals actually precede the patient's death, occurring after the patient's prognosis is rendered hopeless but before there has been a determination of death. This head start is necessary because the technical and social prerequisites to donation take time; the prospects of obtaining and using an organ are increased if steps can be started early. In particular, tissue typing is a time-consuming process, and starting it while the patient is alive increases the chances of placing an organ with a well-matched recipient. In addition, certain treatment practices can improve the prospects that the patient's organs will be in transplantable condition.

Some tension has always existed between the preferred treatment of a head injury and the preferred protocols for protecting organs. Formally, nothing must be done that might compromise the patient's best interests. Practically, there has always been a certain amount of compromise. For example, one standard method of responding to a brain trauma is dehydration to reduce swelling, even though dehydration is not desirable from the point of view of organ protection. Similarly, certain drugs that may be useful for treatment are nephrotoxic. No ethical physician would compromise the treatment of a patient to protect organs for future transplantation, and no neurosurgeon treating a head trauma has the slightest motivation for doing so. However, there is clearly a point at which the physician knows that the patient is doomed; it is at this time that compromises in treatment plans may occur so that manifestly futile and extreme treatments that might endanger vital organs are not undertaken.

Obviously, such considerations arise in the premortem period. However realistic and necessary, they are very sensitive issues for neurosurgeons and are generally not discussed. Yet the incidence of AIDS has increased the need for premortem decision making. AIDS can be transmitted by organ transplantation, and AIDS tests are very time-consuming. OPOs therefore want to run tests before an organ is excised. These tests serve no clinical purpose and do not benefit the patient, but they do potentially help protect recipients and substantially facilitate the procurement process. Knowing the immunological characteristics of the donor early makes finding a suitable recipient much easier.

Declaration of Death and Family Encounters

Most premortem decisions are made cooperatively between the OPO and the nursing staff of the ICU. But physician involvement is also necessary, not just for referral but also for the determination of brain death, made while the heart is still

27

pumping. For the organs of a cadaver to be usable for transplantation, "warm ischemic time"—the period between the cessation of blood flow and the cooling of the organ—must be less than two minutes. This technical necessity requires that the hearts of organ donors be beating (assisted by equipment) when organ removal begins. This precludes declaring death through traditional cardiopulmonary tests. Instead, donors must be declared dead by brain death criteria, as determined by a neurologist or a neurosurgeon. Physicians must also inform the family that death has occurred, even though the heart continues to beat.

Most OPOs look to the ICU medical staff for help in approaching the family of a potential donor. All expect that the staff will have prepared the family for the possibility of donation, and some leave the entire request process in the hospital's hands. A majority, however, prefer to have their own employees request the donation. Handling this encounter is another of the core tasks of organ procurement. As mentioned in Chapter One, the section of the Uniform Anatomical Gift Act that permits a person to will organs without specific family permission is never applied. Organ procurement is done only after the donor's family's permission has been requested and granted.

Logistics

Once death has been declared and permission obtained, the medical procedures to protect the viability of organs can proceed. Donor maintenance, which is largely the responsibility of the ICU nurses, must be as short as an OPO can make it. (Donor maintenance involves monitoring the heart-lung machine, blood electrolytes, and other matters.) Some delay is inevitable while an operating room is arranged and medical teams are assembled, but there are social as well as medical reasons for promptness. Medically, the donor is unstable, as most homeostatic mechanisms die with the brain. Socially, the family is waiting until the end of the process to take possession of the body. If only kidneys are being retrieved, only the local kidney transplant teams must be assembled, and they may have already been alerted. However, if a heart or a liver is involved, a special team may come from a more distant center, and the cold ischemic time (the time between organ removal and transplantation, during which the organ is kept cold) for these organs is short—six to twelve hours. Careful logistical plans must therefore be made to bring the procured organ to the hospital where the recipient waits. Logistical planning is the responsibility of the OPO staff.

Placement

OPOs must also see to it that each donor kidney is used. The local OPO will also have to place any nonrenal organs procured by a local transplant team. If a team from another OPO procured the organs, that OPO is responsible for their use. However, because nonrenal organs must be transplanted so quickly, the recipient of a liver or a heart is generally determined before procurement actually occurs. Once the immunological profile of the kidney is known, the search for a recipient can begin. Surgeons differ about what constitutes a suitable recipient. Many believe that a good match between the donor organ and the recipient's immunological system is essential. Six identified antigens are known to affect the rejection response of a transplant patient; in principle, the larger the number of shared antigens, the greater the likelihood of success (how much greater remains a hotly contested issue). Once an acceptable recipient has been identified, a "cross-match" must be done; this involves mixing sera of the donor and the recipient to see if a reaction occurs. If there is none, the transplant can proceed.

Obtaining a cross-match is a critical step. The immunological system is far more complex than implied by the focus on six antigens, and it is entirely possible that a three- or four-antigen match might also result in a positive cross-match (a cross-match in which a rejection reaction occurs). At the present state of knowledge, no kidney transplant can occur without the physical mixing of specimens from both donor and recipient. This takes time but presents no significant problem if the OPO has a local recipient. Every potential recipient leaves the needed specimens with the local histocompatibility lab, so for locally procured organs, bringing the sera together presents no problem. It is more difficult if the organ is to be sent to another OPO.

If no local surgeon wants to transplant a given kidney, the OPO will export it to another OPO. The national recipient waiting list maintained on computer by the United Network for Organ Sharing (UNOS) provides names of kidney patients; however, until sera from the donor are actually sent to the recipient OPO and tested, it cannot be known if that recipient is in fact suitable. Sending an organ from Boston to Dallas, doing a cross-match in Dallas, and then finding out that the recipient will not do can exhaust the storage life of the kidney.

Professional Education

Although donations are the reasons why OPOs exist, these organizations undertake many other tasks. The referral that starts the donation process is itself the result of prolonged efforts. Almost all organ donors die in intensive care units. As sympathetic to organ procurement as the key medical staff of these ICUs might be, they have other pressing concerns: their job is to save lives, not to salvage organs. OPOs therefore spend much time encouraging doctors and nurses in ICUs to identify potential donors and to inform them accordingly. These efforts range from in-service training sessions to unscheduled visits to the units and personal interviews with key physicians. All of these efforts—in aggregate they exceed the time actually spent procuring organs—are referred to as professional education.

On average, just under 30 percent of the time of an OPO is spent on professional education. Only 25 percent goes to tasks directly needed to procure organs. The remainder is split among organ placement, public education, and routine administration. These percentages have been remarkably constant over the years, although as OPOs have grown and as government involvement has increased, the administrative chores have increased as well. The time spent on maintaining proper records, preparing reports, and complying with paperwork requirements has more than doubled to 10 percent of total time (Prottas, Hecht, and Batten, 1987).

The time spent on professional education reflects its central place in the strategy of organ procurement. It is, in effect, a program of targeted marketing to medical professionals. This activity is so critical that it is the subject of Chapter Four. Successful professional education is the result of a series of tasks, starting with the selection of the best hospitals with which to work. A good source of organ referrals is a hospital with an active trauma unit and a neurosurgeon or a neurologist. In the

31

selected hospitals, nurses in the ICU become the primary marketing target. This reflects their greater accessibility and susceptibility compared to doctors, their greater involvement in the donor maintenance effort, and their generally better rapport with families. Even so, doctors are the final arbiters of access to patients, and they too must be wooed. A good professional education plan is the foundation of success in organ donation.

The National Organ Procurement System

The U.S. organ procurement system is the largest in the world by a substantial margin. The second-largest system, the Eurotransplant Foundation, serving Germany, Austria, and the Benelux nations, is only about 40 percent the size of the American; the French and British national systems are third and fourth in size and together procure one organ for every four procured in the United States. In 1992, the sixty-five agencies in the United States located more than 4,200 donors and worked with almost 5,200 hospitals. Organ procurement has become a sizable industry (Table 2.1).

The OPO system provides very good coverage across the nation. Of the nation's 6,100 acute care hospitals, over 80 percent are associated with an OPO. In this context, it is worth noting that only 31 percent of hospitals served by OPOs actually provided a donor in 1986. The size of the waiting list is also worth noting: more than twenty-three thousand people were waiting for a kidney transplant in 1992.

The size of the procurement system is reflected in the scale of its activities. More than 4,200 cadaveric organ donors in 1991 provided almost 13,000 transplantable organs: 7,800 kidneys

Table 2.1. Scale of the National Organ Procurement System.

	1982	1986	1991
Number of active OPOs	82	100	68
Population served (millions)	219.4	222.8	248.2
Hospitals served	2,500	4,450	5,137
Hospitals supplying donors	950	1,350	—[a]
Total kidney waiting list	6,000	11,300	21,090
Number of donors	—[b]	4,100	4,300
Number of kidneys	5,070	7,740	7,641
Number of referrals	5,970	11,000	13,200

[a]Not available.
[b]Figures not gathered.
Source: Adapted from Prottas, 1982, 1987; General Accounting Office, 1992.

(2,200 more came from living donors), 2,100 hearts, and 3,000 livers. Finally, the number of referrals is an important measure because it reflects the level of cooperation of medical professionals. In 1992, more than thirteen thousand calls were made to OPOs to report potential donors.

The organ procurement system is impressive not only for its actual size but also for its rate of growth. As Table 2.1 shows, there was very substantial growth in all areas except for the total population served between 1982 and 1986. By 1982, the system had grown to cover virtually the entire nation, but in the next four years, the number of hospitals served increased by almost 80 percent, the number of kidneys procured by almost 37 percent, and the number of referrals by about 85 percent.

Since 1986, a different pattern has emerged, one of very little growth. In part this reflects the maturing of the organ procurement system in the late 1980s. Almost all parts of the country were being served by this time, and most suitable hospitals had already been drawn into the referral net. The number of OPOs decreased to sixty-eight in 1991 due to consolidation and the weeding out of inactive or marginal organizations. Referrals continued to rise slightly, thanks in part to required request laws, and the waiting list for organs increased substantially. This last increase reflects both success and failure. Improved graft survival rates have made kidney transplantation a more attractive treatment option, and so patients and physicians have sought it more frequently. Unfortunately, organ procurement success has not kept pace either with this increased demand or with prior rates of increase. Since 1986, the number of organ donors in the United States has been stable at about 4,100 to 4,200. From 1986 to 1989, there was no increase in the number of cadaveric kidney transplants (between 7,000 and 7,100); 1990 saw an increase to 7,700, but 1992 saw no improvement on that number. During the years 1986–1992, the number of kidney transplants increased only about 10 percent. This plateauing of organ supply has become one of the basic policy and organizational questions facing the nation's organ procurement system.

Donor Population

Table 2.2 shows the characteristics of the donor population during the 1980s. It has been remarkably stable. The minor changes in the percentage of donors from the various racial groups are insignificant. Indeed, the table calls into question the once accepted fact that African-Americans donate organs less frequently than whites. Although the figures on donor race are only estimates, they indicate that more blacks participate than previously thought. Because a small number of OPOs with a large percentage of black donors (1986 data only) may distort the

Table 2.2. Donor Characteristics.[a]

	1982	1986	1989–1990
Donors			
White	86.2	84.2	80.8
Black	8.8	9.7	9.5
Hispanic	4.6	5.5	7.0
Asian and other	0.5	0.5	1.3
Potential donors granting permission	71.5	71.4	59.5
Donors granting permission for multiorgan donation	—[b]	56.6	75.6

[a]All figures are percentages.
[b]Not available.
Source: Adapted from United Network for Organ Sharing, 1991b; General Accounting Office, 1992.

average, the median percentage (7.0) of black donors may be a more accurate measure. Even 7 percent is significant and shows that black Americans are participating in organ donation in considerable numbers. Data gathered in 1990 from a representative sample of OPOs indicate that the percentage of African-American donors has remained around 9 percent and that of Hispanic donors has increased to about 7 percent. Both these numbers are below these groups' share in the general population, but neither supports the contention that racial or ethnic minority groups donate at sharply lower rates than the rest of the population.

One characteristic that has changed dramatically is the percentage of donors who agree to donate more than one organ. This is almost certainly a function of the fact that far more OPOs are now trying to procure hearts and livers as well as kidneys. It also explains how the very rapid increase in the number of nonrenal transplants has been possible. In 1986, over half of all kidney donors also donated another organ; by 1990, that figure had risen to 76 percent.

Because donor criteria for nonrenal organs is more stringent than for kidney donors, we have reached the end of the dramatic upturn in nonrenal transplants. When all suitable kidney donors are donating other organs as well, the increase in non-renal transplants will be tied to improvements in the ability to locate donors—just as increases in kidney transplants have always been. Once again the natural constraint on transplants—donor supply—will come into play. Nevertheless, it is a triumph of flexibility and determination on the part of the organ procurement system that it adapted to the demand for nonrenal organs so quickly and successfully. It is also indicative of the character of organ donor families that they quickly agreed to the expanded requests made of them.

Structure and Control

The organization and structure of the organ procurement system have undergone substantial changes as the scale of operations has expanded. Independent OPOs now dominate, and whereas in the early 1980s, most OPOs served only a single transplant center, now about 80 percent of them serve more than one hospital. A substantial number of members who are not transplant surgeons must now sit on all OPO boards of directors. In 1986, only 22 percent of OPOs had any board of directors at all; the remainder were essentially under the direct control of a single transplant surgeon. At that time, the interagency organ sharing system was voluntary, and organs were shared on an informal and ad hoc basis, as Chapter Five will discuss. The organ procurement system now has a highly developed and very powerful national framework.

Nevertheless, OPOs are still dominated by transplant surgeons, and the national organ sharing system too is largely in their hands. The growth of the organ procurement system since 1982 and its increased professionalism have increased the independence of OPO nonmedical staff, and government intervention has boosted the role of the lay public over OPO practice. But transplant surgeons continue to dominate for a number of reasons. First of all, donor maintenance and selection, tissue typing, and the location of suitable recipients are all technical activities in which policies cannot be set without the expertise of the transplant community. Second, no outsider has as continuous and passionate an interest in the practice of OPOs as transplant surgeons do. All of the "raw material" essential to the practice of their profession comes from OPOs: their professional success, reputation, status, and income depend on the quantity and quality of the donated organs. The desire of these surgeons to be their own directors is therefore very strong; supported by their necessary technical knowledge and the status and prestige of their calling, it ensures their effective domination of local OPOs.

Effectiveness in Organ Procurement

The American organ procurement system locates and obtains organs with exceptional efficacy. The best measure of success is the number of kidneys procured on a per capita basis. In 1982, the system procured 18.5 kidneys per million population. In contrast, the Eurotransplant Foundation procured only 15.9 per million, and the other major European organ procurement systems, in Great Britain and France, did not do even that well (Prottas, 1985). In organ procurement, the American genius for fragmentation, heterogeneity, and local-level association has proved itself exceptionally appropriate.

The development of the position of organ procurement coordinator is a second factor contributing to the American success. Nationally, some four hundred organ procurement coordinators are at work. Their role is essentially that of a sales representative, marketing professional education and managing the logistics of the organ procurement process. This role was not nearly so well developed in Europe in the early 1980s. Only the Netherlands operated in a comparable way—and only the Netherlands had comparable success.

Since the mid 1980s, we have seen a convergence of practices and level of success between Europe and the United States in terms of organ procurement. The technical tasks in organ procurement are, of course, the same in any part of the world. North America and Europe are so culturally similar that many of the social issues regarding families and medical professionals are also the same. Over the past decade, the American practice of using transplant coordinators and actively engaging in hospital development has spread throughout Europe (just as the development of the national Organ Procurement and Transplantation Network, to be discussed in Chapter Five, approximates European organ sharing systems). As a result, success rates throughout the Atlantic community have climbed and converged. In 1990, U.S. OPOs procured about 32 kidneys per million population served. This is higher than the rates found in Scandinavia, Spain, and the United Kingdom and lower than the rates obtained in France and in the Eurotransplant service area (United Network for Organ Sharing, 1992).

The importance of coordinators and of the community-based nature of the OPOs is consistent. The latter reflects the integration of organ procurement and local medical institutions; the former, the divergence of organ procurement from health care provision. The organ procurement coordinator's role reflects the professionalization of organ procurement in the United States or at least the specialization of that role. This specialization has other aspects: the primacy of nonmedical skills in OPOs (marketing skills in particular), the historical superiority of independent organ procurement organizations (IOPOs), and the positive relationship between the scale of an OPO's activities and its effectiveness. Each of these factors can most clearly be seen when the effectiveness of different OPOs in the United States is compared.

Success at Organ Procurement

The organ procurement system has shown itself to be capable of great flexibility and learning, as is evident from its rapid growth and effectiveness during the mid 1980s and especially its continuing response to the new demands of nonrenal transplantation. In 1986, the average OPO was more effective than the best 10 percent of OPOs in 1982! Much of this change reflects the diffusion and acceptance of successful organizational technologies for organ procurement. In particular, procurement moved away from the model of a medical supply service to that of a marketing and sales organization. This distancing between the procurer and the transplant hospital is characteristic of independent organ procurement organizations, and their larger

39

scale offered them not only increased expertise but also increased independence. As a result, the ratio of independent to hospital OPOs has shifted.

In 1982, only about a third of OPOs were independently organized; in 1986, about half were; by 1990, the figure had increased to 75 percent. Overall, the system has shifted in operational patterns and orientation in the directions traditionally associated with IOPOs so that there are now clear signs of convergence.

Independent and hospital OPOs have so converged that this structural factor, once critical, no longer explains many of the differences found among the OPOs. On the other hand, organizational size has come to be more important. The continued importance of referrals shows that professional education programs remain the key to organ procurement success. Perhaps the most striking change in recent years is the new importance of permission rates. In 1982, differences in organizational effectiveness were so great that the percentage of families granting permission had no effect on procurement outcomes. In fact, the poorer OPOs had higher permission rates than the better ones, primarily because they were so ineffective at locating donors in the first place that they encountered only families already strongly motivated to donate. By 1986, the professionalism and competence of OPOs had grown so that their ability to persuade families mattered.

Overall, the change in the production function of OPOs reflects the new maturity of the organ procurement system, in which the core tasks of the process are well understood and widely implemented. Success is now a function of actual effectiveness at performing the key tasks—with the important exception of the impact of organizational size. As the size of an organ procurement organization has a direct effect on its ability to succeed at its key tasks, so the growth of the organ procurement system itself has played a role in its increased effectiveness.

The nature of the connection between size and effectiveness is not obscure. Larger agencies have two important advantages over smaller ones. First, they can more easily select the hospitals with which to work, and not all hospitals are equally good sources of donors. They differ both in terms of the kinds and numbers of patients they treat and in the attitudes of their key staff. A large OPO serving numerous hospitals can allocate its resources where the most return in terms of hospital cooperation can be obtained. In addition, a larger OPO can support the staff necessary to maintain its professional education effort in the face of the unpredictable and unavoidable demands of donor calls. OPOs are subject to two kinds of demands that differ in intensity and time frame. Actual donor calls are imperative and, indeed, the raison d'être of the agency. But education and marketing efforts are the long-term investment that will define the ultimate success of the organization. A small OPO cannot always maintain its education program in the face of more immediate demands, making its efforts in this area less predictable and less systematic. Thus a smaller OPO is forced into a reactive stance.

The practical question now becomes, at what point is an OPO too small? Some data indicate that organizations with fewer than fifty or so donors a year face a relatively difficult task ensuring adequate professional education time. However, there is no evidence that very large agencies have any inherent advantage over those procuring between fifty and one hundred donors.

Flat National Supply

Why organ supply has been relatively stable since 1986 is not clear. In part it may reflect the maturation of the system itself. By the mid 1980s, the key elements of OPO success were widely understood, and the organizations' practices were converging toward a universal standard. It might be thought, therefore, that present procurement rates are the best obtainable given present organizational knowledge and policy. However, we still find substantial differences among OPOs in terms of organs procured per capita. Though these differences are less extreme than they were in the early 1980s (when the best OPO procured almost ten times as many organs per capita as the worst), they are still substantial (Evans, Orrans, and Uscher, 1992). It may be that the least effective OPOs are so resistant to change that improvement through the spread of standardized best practices is at a standstill and will remain so unless ineffective OPOs come under external pressures to change.

It is also possible that more basic factors are at work. The organ procurement system is procuring more organs per capita than it did a decade ago, and it is certain that many more potential donors still exist. But there is reason to believe that the actual *pool* of donors is decreasing (Nathan and others, 1991). Seat belt laws, higher minimum drinking age, and enforcement of drunk driving laws have all decreased the number of traffic fatalities in the United States. In 1986, perhaps 45 percent of all organ donors died as a result of motor vehicle accidents; in 1990, only 25 percent did (United Network for Organ Sharing, 1991b). Considering that around a third of all potential donors actually donate, a smaller pool increases the challenge facing OPOs. The first third (or quarter or whatever) of potential donors are certainly more easily obtained than the remainder. Each increment requires more effort, as it means identifying less obviously suitable donors and/or persuading less obviously supportive families. It may be that a flat national supply actually reflects increasing organ procurement effectiveness in the context of a diminishing potential donor pool.

In summation, it is not clear how much of the stagnation in organ supply is due to organizational factors within the organ procurement system and how much is due to broader factors. Undoubtedly, some of the problem is organizational and can be dealt with by operational improvement. However, prolonged stagnation of organ supply has also raised the possibility that public action is needed, action that might alter the present system of organ procurement in various ways, including the introduction of market incentives and the alteration of the relationship between hospitals and organ procurement organizations to allow the latter better access to patient information.

Public Policies and the Organ Procurement System

There has been substantial change in recent years in the role of public policy in organ procurement. Congress has been at the forefront of pressing for the socialization of the organ procurement system. Public intervention has occurred on several levels. As noted, there was the rapid and almost universal enactment of required request laws. It is impossible to overstate the ethical revolution implied by these laws. Congress and virtually every state have said, in effect, that the medical profession's assistance in organ procurement is obligatory. The clear implication is that organ donation is primarily a social issue, legitimately under the direct purview of public bodies, and not solely a medical question subject to the professional judgment and ethics of physicians.

Government Intervention

According to the other systemwide interventions enacted in the National Organ Transplantation Act of 1984 and as part of the Omnibus Budget Reconciliation Act (OBRA) of 1986, the nation's entire organ procurement system comes under the control of the secretary of Health and Human Services. First, the secretary, acting through the Health Care Financing Administration (HCFA), has the right and obligation to specify the service areas of each OPO. In the past, an OPO could lay claim to any area it chose, limited only by the willingness of hospitals to refer donors and competition from other nearby OPOs. Service areas were informal and frequently overlapped. The rules for OPO certification were minimal and contained no requirement pertaining to the location of donor hospitals. As a result, in many places, several OPOs might be servicing a single area, and many OPOs might claim to be servicing overlapping areas.

OBRA, enacted in 1986, required that the secretary of Health and Human Services end this laissez-faire system. Under this law, the secretary was obliged to grant exclusive franchises to OPOs. Every OPO that wished to operate had to submit to the HCFA a plan specifying its service area in detail, along with documentation showing that 75 percent of hospitals in that area had agreed to refer organs to the OPO. In addition, the service areas had to have certain characteristics: they had to be exclusive, no other OPO could claim any part of another's, they had to include all of a metropolitan area or none (only one franchise to a city), and they had to be large (2.5 million people and/or fifty potential donors was the working minimum). In the case of competing claims, the federal government would decide who could procure organs and who could not. No organ procured by an unfranchised OPO would be paid for, and, even more important, any hospital doing transplants with such an organ could be totally excluded from the Medicare system.

In addition, the secretary was given the responsibility of monitoring OPO performance over time. This too was a radical break from past practices. Prior to 1988 (when the 1986 law was implemented), once an OPO was given a provider number, its subsequent performance was irrelevant—in fact, several OPOs had held provider numbers for a decade without procuring a single organ! Now HCFA must recertify each OPO every two years, on the basis of performance standards. This means that it is no longer sufficient merely to have specified personnel and organizational characteristics. It is necessary to procure a certain number of organs on a per capita basis and to ensure the transplantation of a certain number of kidneys per million population served. Failure to meet these performance standards can lead to decertification and the transfer of the franchise to another organization.

Before 1986, the federal government paid for 90 percent of all the costs of organ procurement in the United States and had no legal right to interfere in the system that generated those costs. Since then, the government's share of organ procurement costs has dropped to about 65 percent (due to the increase in nonrenal transplants), and it has assumed the responsibility for structuring, monitoring, and evaluating the entire system.

Beyond its extensive direct control of the system, the federal government also has powerful indirect control via the national Organ Procurement and Transplantation Network. Congress has required that all OPOs and transplant hospitals be members of that organization before being permitted to do any organ transplantation or procurement. The Network has a large number of membership rules regarding policies and operational standards, including requirements that transplant hospitals have certain kinds of staff and do certain minimum numbers of transplants. Health and Human Services has assumed responsibility for reviewing the Network's membership requirements and has final approval on all its rules. This not only reinforces its immense control over the OPO system, but it also extends that control directly to transplant hospitals. By 1988, the federal government had developed the legal and organizational tools needed to assume effective control over the American system of organ procurement and transplantation.

Public Practice

In fact, the federal bureaucracy has taken a timid approach in "franchising" OPOs. It has interpreted the law in ways that were calculated to interfere the least with the status quo. For example, although an OPO must have agreements with 75 percent of hospitals in its service area, any hospital may deal with any OPO, even if that hospital is not in its designated service area. This nullifies the concept of noncompeting service areas, as adjacent OPOs can freely operate in each other's areas. Also, no OPO has been refused certification by HCFA, despite some rather transparent and pro forma "consolidations" of previously competing OPOs.

In 1990, the average OPO procured more than 30 kidneys per million population served. HCFA required 21 per million— 30 percent less than the average! HCFA rules also define an acceptable wastage rate (percentage of organs procured that are not actually used) of about 14 percent, and this is far above the present national average of 5 to 7 percent. HCFA's standards, like its certification process, appear designed to avoid rather than solidify the public's new role in organ procurement. When the recertification process threatened to disqualify a number of OPOs in 1990, HCFA first delayed application of the law and then obtained new authority to rewrite certification rules. Regulations have still not been promulgated, and so for nearly a decade, no OPO has been evaluated, much less found to have failed to meet minimal performance standards.

In fact, HCFA has taken an aggressive stand in only one area: limiting Network intervention on certification matters. As we shall see, the national Network cannot be understood as an enemy of the status quo in transplantation, but it did promulgate more rigorous requirements for the membership of hospitals than HCFA promulgated for the certification of transplant programs. Since membership in the Network is as essential to a transplant program as certification by the government, some hospitals objected to the Network's rules, and HCFA acted vigorously to force the Network to modify its requirements. HCFA then went on to ensure that in future conflicts, the secretary of Health and Human Services would prevail.

If we could attribute strategy to the Department of Health and Human Services, it might be that the federal government has asserted the primacy of public institutions over the medical profession in organ transplantation while carefully declining to exercise that primacy. Congress decided, with the support of most state governments and the acquiescence of the transplant community, that public oversight of this area is needed. The Reagan and Bush administrations found that prospect distasteful, and the bureaucracy finds it daunting; both reactions advise delay and minimalism. In this, as in so many other aspects of public transplantation policy, we are in a time of basic change in principle and minimal change in practice. In Chapter Five we will see that this pattern continues in the key area of organ distribution.

3

The Public
and Organ Donation

ORGAN PROCUREMENT DEPENDS on people—but not on all people because the opportunity and catastrophe of giving can only occur to people who find themselves caught in a complex web of tragedy, technology, and kindness. The complexity is exacerbated by the irreducible variety of the human actors— by their feelings about death, family relations, religion, and philosophy and by their understanding and attitude toward some of the most advanced and esoteric medical technologies. In this chapter, we will examine the role of the public in organ donation and how that role is defined by the structure of the organ procurement process. We will consider the heterogeneity of the giving public, both in terms of demographic and social factors and in terms of knowledge and beliefs. We are concerned with who can give, who will give, and why.

The Principle of Giving

It is not fashionable to speak of the power of altruism or the inspirational nature of generosity, but organ transplantation rests wholly on altruism and generosity. To understand how altruism translates into organ donation, it is necessary to understand the principles that define the role of the public in the donation process. First, donation is voluntary. The core principle of our donation system is that disposal of the body of the deceased is a private decision in which public involvement is inappropriate. The donation decision is not a matter of public policy; however, the factors that may motivate that decision are. More precisely, public policy spells out what may *not* motivate donation; for example, organ donation may not be compensated—the voluntary decision to donate must be based on altruistic motives; otherwise, it is not permitted. Altruism is thus a second basic principle of organ donation. Finally, it is necessary to understand whose voluntarism and altruism are involved: the families of donors.

Families are the decision-making unit in organ donation. The law vests that right in the donors themselves, to be exercised by a donor card, but in practice it is exercised by mothers, fathers, children and siblings. Personal willingness to donate one's own organs tells us something about an individual's kindness but very little about the actual supply of organs. The real criterion is the willingness to donate the organs of a loved one. The donation decision is therefore not an individual one but a familial one.

Our system of organ procurement has been called "assisted voluntarism" (Caplan and Welvang, 1989), which means that a donor family usually does not initiate the donation process but is first approached by organ procurement specialists. If the family agrees, it is mandatory that its permission be explicit and in writing.

Another model of the public's role exists. Several European countries have "presumed consent" laws. Under these laws, "passive voluntarism" is permitted. Donor families may refuse organ donation, but to do so they must actively state an objection.

In these nations, organ procurement can go forward without obtaining the explicit permission of the family, which is simply presumed.

Although there is no widespread support for this sort of voluntarism in organ procurement in the United States, twenty-three states do operate cornea donation under a presumed consent system. These "medical examiner laws" allow the removal of corneas from cadavers without the explicit permission of next of kin. (In fact, these laws differ one from the other in many ways. Some require no family notification at all; in others, a pro forma effort at obtaining permission is mandated; and still others require a "good faith" effort. In all cases, if the family cannot be contacted, the medical examiner may give permission to proceed without the family (Aiken-O'Neill, 1992.) These laws operate quite effectively and without serious public objection or awareness. Often families don't even know that the procedure is being performed. Under these presumed consent laws, cornea donation remains voluntary but is "less voluntary" than organ donation.

As a result, cornea donation is perhaps less altruistic but just as uncompensated as other organ donations. The rule is that no remuneration be given for any donation, a practice that antedates the passage of federal law and extends beyond its requirements. Not only is no payment made, but organ procurement organizations will assume only costs that result directly from organ procurement activities, such as lab tests and operating room time. What then motivates donors? In the midst of a major life tragedy and for no reward but kindness itself, 60 to 70 percent of the American public agrees to help a stranger.

The Context of Giving

The archetypical organ donor is a young man who is in an auto accident and ultimately dies of his injuries. Such a victim first arrives at an emergency room and, if he survives initial medical encounters, is transferred to an intensive care unit. In many cases, this will be a neurological ICU, as most organ donors succumb to damage to the central nervous system. That is why auto accident, gunshot wound to the head, and cerebral vascular accident (stroke) are the primary diagnoses that presage organ donation. In such a case, a neurophysician, often a neurosurgeon, is called in and assumes much of the responsibility for care. When the doctor or the ICU nurse comes to the realization that the patient cannot live and informs an organ procurement organization that the dying patient could be a suitable organ donor, the focus begins to shift from the patient and technical concerns to the family and emotional ones. When asked to grant permission for the removal of their kin's organs, between 60 and 70 percent of all families accede. This is the central truth of organ donation. Some may speak of the "kindness of strangers" with irony, but nobody in organ procurement does.

However, not all people are asked. Many—and no one knows just how many—are never approached. This failure to ask is a primary impediment to increasing organ supply. Nevertheless, it is arguable that those asked are a select population and that citing the 60 to 70 percent who say yes overestimates the actual willingness of the public to give (Nathan and others, 1991; Prottas and Batten, 1991b). There remain the 30 to 40 percent who refuse. Therefore, at least two initial questions have to be addressed: what proportion of the public is willing to donate, and how do people who are willing differ from those who are not? After that comes the more practical question of what, if anything, can be done to persuade the unwilling to reconsider.

Willingness to Donate: Changes in Time and Place

Public attitudes toward organ donation have changed over the past ten or fifteen years, and there are differences among Atlantic community nations in terms of these attitudes. The changes in attitude, however, have been far less striking than the changes in the transplantation process itself, and overall, the continuity and similarity are more striking than change and difference. Some of the earliest inquiries into public attitudes toward organ donation are more than twenty-five years old and antedate the widespread application of the technical procedures used today. In 1968, the Gallup Organization conducted a poll on attitudes toward organ donation and reported that 70 percent of respondents would consider donating their own organs. This was four years before the passage of the End-Stage Renal Disease Act and the start of widespread organ transplantation. Clearly, the responses obtained by Gallup reflected a general willingness of people to be of help and were not based on any firm knowledge of the need for or effectiveness of that help.

The 1968 survey was the beginning of a long chain of research into public attitudes toward organ donation. This work has suffered from several shortcomings, including poorly conceived questions, poor sample selection, and inadequate sample size. Often the research has been funded by groups with as much interest in making a point as in determining a fact.

Nevertheless, results have been reasonably consistent. In surveys conducted in different parts of the country over a period of nineteen years, it was found that between 66 and 78 percent of respondents supported organ donation and would consider authorizing the use of a relative's organ (Cleveland, 1975; Gallup Organization, 1983, 1985). Other consistencies also appear. Willingness is high, communication low: though 70 percent of the population express support, only about 30 percent have discussed the matter. Social factors have always correlated highly with willingness to donate. All of the early work that examined the issue found that race and class were strongly associated with support of organ donation. Whites were more supportive than blacks, and the better-educated and wealthier were more supportive than the less educated and poorer. Regional and religious factors were not at all decisive, and age was only marginally significant.

Data from other nations are scant, but where they exist, they tend to show that the attitudes of Western Europeans are very similar to those of Americans. Data from the United Kingdom from around the time of most U.S. studies show that 68 percent of respondents would grant permission for an organ donation, but in contrast to equivalent U.S. data, almost 58 percent of the population had discussed donation with their families (Moore, Clarse, Lewis, and Malhet, 1976). Recent data from Canada and Sweden are also comparable with recent American data (Stiller, 1984; Bergstrom and Gabel, 1991). The Canadian work indicates that 78 percent of the population would grant permission for an organ donation.

The Swedish findings differ in a way that highlights an important shortcoming of most surveys on public attitudes toward organ donation. Only 45 percent of Swedish respondents stated their willingness to permit the donation of a relative's organs *when that relative had not made his or her own wishes known.* The question has rarely been phrased like this, yet this is the most useful question to ask. When 70 percent of respondents say that they would permit an organ donation, the question they are responding to does not specify anything about the donor's personal preferences. This oversight exaggerates support for organ donation. More than 90 percent of people say they will honor a relative's wish to donate. Therefore, combining people acting on instructions and people acting on their own in a single statistic double-counts many yes responses.

If consistency in public attitudes is broad, is it deep? Attitudes toward organ donation are not adequately represented by an answer to a single question. To understand variations (or their absence) among the publics polled, it is necessary to examine more closely the building blocks of public support.

Key Public Attitudes in Organ Donation

The public is extremely supportive of organ donation (see Table 3.1): 90 percent of respondents surveyed say they strongly approve of it. An almost equally high number believe that organ donation can help a family deal with the grief of bereavement.

Great willingness is also expressed to participate in the donation process—almost three-quarters of respondents reacted positively. Willingness to donate one's own organs is relevant to actual donation, however, only if that decision is communicated to one's family. Organ donors are clearly not in a position to state preferences, and only a minority of Americans have discussed this matter with their families. Family attitudes about

Table 3.1. General Support for Organ Donation.

Statement	Percentage of Respondents Agreeing
I strongly approve of organ donation.	90
Organ donation helps with grief.	81
I have discussed organ donation with my family.	46
I would donate my own organs.	72
I would donate the organs of a relative who had not discussed the issue.	53
I would donate the organs of a relative who was known to be brain-dead.	78
If my relative had stated a willingness to be an organ donor, I'd give permission.	94

Source: Adapted from Prottas and Batten, 1991b.

donation are thus more immediately important: slightly more than half of respondents (53 percent) expressed unequivocal willingness; an additional 25 percent (for a total of 78 percent) said yes after the brain death of their kin was made an explicit part of the question. Finally, about 20 percent of the public is strongly resistant to organ donation. Half of these people are so hostile that they would block a donation that they knew the deceased would have supported.

No important differences have been noted regarding willingness to donate by organ involved. Attitudes toward tissue donation were not tested, but among people who would permit donation, more than 90 percent were willing to donate any of the commonly transplanted vascularized organs.

Knowledge of the details of organ transplantation and donation is not as universal as support for them (see Table 3.2). Most of the public has heard of organ donation cards, but few people have signed them; many believe that a central registry

Table 3.2. Knowledge Among the Public.

Statement	Percentage of Respondents Agreeing
I have heard of donor cards.	83
I have signed a donor card.	20[a]
A central file of card signers exists.	25
Once you sign a card, you can't change your mind.	6
The donor must permit a donation.	82
The family must permit a donation.	62
A doctor can permit a donation.	6
Kidney transplantation is still experimental.	30
Heart transplantation is still experimental.	55
Liver transplantation is still experimental.	49
The public is well informed about organ transplantation.	47

[a]A 1992 survey by the National Kidney Foundation found that 33 percent of respondents said that they had signed donor cards.

Source: Adapted from Gallup Organization, 1985; Prottas and Batten, 1991b.

exists for storing lists of those who have signed a card. In addition, the belief is widespread that the donor must personally give permission; only 60 percent understand that families must do so. Finally, a large percentage of the public erroneously believes that well-established transplantation procedures, especially heart transplants, are still experimental.

The public does not consider itself very well informed about organ transplantation, but the data can be read in different ways. Certainly, none of the Gallup poll data imply sophisticated or broad knowledge about transplantation or organ donation, but the general outlines of the process and the system do seem to be understood. Most people know that it is a voluntary system. Most have heard of brain death (82 percent) and seem to have at least a general idea that it means that the brain has stopped functioning. The major lesson to be drawn from the gap between support and knowledge is that the importance of knowledge is overestimated. The one-year graft survival of a heart transplant is 80 percent; even though 55 percent of people still believe it to be an experimental procedure, they are nevertheless willing to donate. There may be some minimum level of understanding that must be reached to ensure public support for organ donation, but it is clear that we have surpassed that level. It is also clear—the earlier discussions of families of donors reinforce this—that educators and professionals grossly overestimate the amount and accuracy of knowledge the public needs.

Social Bases of Support

Support for organ donation and willingness to donate are not evenly distributed across the American population, but certain classic demographic variables do not have much relevance. For example, we find no significant differences between regions of the country or even among rural, urban, and suburban Americans.

Similarly, there are few differences among religious groups, and all major religions support organ donation. With only minor exceptions, religious beliefs do not affect attitudes toward organ donation. Nor does the reported intensity of religious commitment.

If region and religion do not matter at all, age and sex matter almost as little. Women are more likely than men to believe that a donation helps the family deal with its grief and tends to diminish the pain of loss. However, these attitudes do not translate into greater overall support or willingness to donate. The effect of age is more complex. Older people are less willing to donate their own organs (perhaps because they understand that they are less suitable) and are also somewhat more willing to impose their preferences regarding donation on deceased relatives—that is, they are less willing to follow the directives of the deceased. Beyond this, they express levels of support and willingness comparable to those of younger Americans. Only in policy preferences is there any sign of generational differences. Older respondents are less willing to support changes in present donation policy (Prottas and Batten, 1986b). They are significantly less supportive of *any* policy innovations that would provide incentives to organ donation, from tax credits to direct cash payments—as the National Kidney Foundation found again in 1992. They are even less supportive of non-incentive-based innovations such as required request laws. Americans over the age of fifty-five appear to be strongly committed to giving in general and to the present structure of giving in particular.

This unanimity does not extend to race and social class (as measured by education and income), which are strongly and independently associated with almost all attitudes toward organ donation. As Table 3.3 shows, black Americans are less supportive of organ donation than white Americans on every question asked. These differences are statistically significant in almost every case.

There are several traditional ways of measuring social class, and none is without shortcomings. Income and education are the two measures used most often. Both are adequate, if rough, measures of social class. Table 3.4 displays attitudes by education level. (The results by income do not differ in important ways.)

Education has an important impact on attitudes, although not with the consistency of race. However, in the key areas

Table 3.3. Support for Organ Donation by Race.

Statement	Percentage of Respondents Agreeing	
	Whites	Blacks
I strongly approve of organ donation.	91	79*
Organ donation helps with grief.	81	74
I have discussed organ donation with my family.	48	21*
I would donate my own organs.	74	51*
I would donate the organs of a relative who had not discussed the issue.	55	37*
I would donate the organs of a relative who was known to be brain-dead.	79	58*
If my relative had stated a willingness to be an organ donor, I'd give permission.	94	85*

*Difference is statistically significant.
Source: Prottas and Batten, 1986b. Used by permission.

of family discussion, personal willingness, and willingness to donate the organs of a relative, education matters.

Both class and race also matter with regard to attitudes toward changes in organ procurement policy. On all of the policy questions asked, with the exception of support for public education efforts, black respondents were more willing to see changes in policy. In each case, they were more supportive of the introduction of incentives into the donation process. They were also more supportive of presumed consent laws but not of required request laws. We find essentially the same pattern by education level. The less educated are more interested in incentives but do not differ greatly on non-incentive-based changes, such as more public education or required request laws.

These findings—which hold for virtually all the surveys done in the past twenty years—are not surprising. African-Americans

Table 3.4. Support for Organ Donation by Education Level.

Statement	Percentage of Respondents Agreeing		
	High School Graduates	People with Some College	College Graduates
I strongly approve of organ donation.	89	88	92
Organ donation helps with grief.	83	77	81
I have discussed organ donation with my family.	38	51	58*
I would donate my own organs.	66	78	79*
I would donate the organs of a relative who had not discussed the issue.	50	53	59*
I would donate the organs of a relative who was known to be brain-dead.	74	80	82*
If my relative had stated a willingness to be an organ donor, I'd give permission.	93	94	95

*Differences are statistically significant.
Source: Prottas and Batten, 1986b. Used by permission.

and the less educated have not committed themselves to organ donation as strongly as better-educated or white Americans have and are therefore more willing to accept changes in the present way of doing things.

Finally, it is important to note that *both* race and class matter, independently, in organ donation attitudes. This was important to determine because race and education are themselves closely correlated in the United States. We examined the separate effects of these two variables using analysis of variance techniques, and in all cases, each had an effect separate from the other. Moreover, in each case, the effect of race was substantially greater than that of education. On organ donation issues, black and white Americans are divided (Prottas and Batten, 1986b).

Attitude Differences Among Americans

Racial and class differences among Americans are strongly related to attitudinal differences, and these relationships affect the role the public plays in the transplantation system. But the actual differences in the attitudes themselves are also important. They directly measure the degree of support the organ procurement system can count on from the public and, perhaps, the kinds of adjustments that might increase that support.

It is possible to begin to delineate the attitudinal segmentation of Americans with regard to organ donation. The Battelle Institute made an initial attempt and found that about 19 percent of the public is "truly unwilling" to donate (Manninen and Evans, 1985). More detailed work at Brandeis University has allowed a more precise differentiation. About 52 percent of Americans are willing to permit the donation of a relative's organs without any knowledge of the deceased's preferences. (This is the actual situation in the vast majority of donations.) Another 29 percent say they would not donate when the simple question of willingness to donate is asked but change their minds after it is made clear that their relative is brain-dead, even though they still did not have any information about that person's preference. The final 19 percent are adamantly opposed to donation and will not give permission under any circumstances. It is the middle 29 percent that are of most concern. This group is persuadable—neither so committed that persuasion is redundant nor so hostile that it is futile (Prottas and Batten, 1991b).

The primary utility of these attitudinal categories is that they allow the development of sensible message content in public education. Two principles ought to guide a public education plan. First, no changes should be pursued that undermine the support of the core constituency, those Americans already willing to donate. Survey data show that a firm base of willingness already exists, so a policy that abandons that base is certain to lead to a decrease in overall support and donation. Second, it is neither possible nor altogether appropriate to try to change the views of the truly unwilling. As a practical matter, people in this segment are the hardest to persuade because their opposition will not be lightly surrendered. Furthermore, some base their views on ethical standards that public agencies have little right to question or undermine. It is doubtful that any public education effort could much affect them, and there is no sound argument for trying. Policy changes and public appeals should therefore concentrate on the 29 percent of Americans who are not willing to donate but might be persuaded to change their minds, so long as these changes and appeals do not alienate the 52 percent who are already firmly convinced. To achieve this, we must understand why people are willing or hesitant to permit donation.

Motives of Givers

If the core support of the donation process is not to be alienated, we must not make changes or frame appeals that are inconsistent with their outlook. The reasons given by supporters of organ donation for their willingness to donate fall into two general categories. The first centers on the benefits to others, cited by more than 88 percent of respondents. The second major reason, cited by almost 65 percent, is not wanting to see usable organs go to waste. Both of these reasons refer to a desire to use organ donation as a way to help others. However, the third and fourth most important reasons have to do with ameliorating the tragedy the respondents faced. Sixty percent say that making something positive come out of the death of their relative is a very important reason for their support; about 40 percent say that the wish to have part of their relative live on is a very important motivation. These answers are all essentially altruistic. The desire to help others obviously predominates in organ donation decision making and also leads many people to seek comfort in generosity rather than in some other way.

There are few racial differences in motivation among people committed to organ donation, although a smaller percentage of blacks is unambiguously committed to donation than whites. The only statistically significant difference between the races involves donation as a way of having the relative live on, with black respondents feeling more strongly about this than whites.

Motives for Refusal

The most important reason given by respondents who express an unwillingness to donate is the wish to avoid prolonging the suffering of their kin (see Table 3.5). Family concerns are the next most important reason for refusal—that is, many believe that some other family member would object. Following in importance is a sense that donation is somehow difficult and complicated and, most disturbing, a fear that doctors would withhold treatment needed by a patient whose family had agreed to organ donation.

Table 3.5. Reasons for Not Donating Organs.

| | Percentage of Respondents Calling Reason "Very Important" | |
Reason	Persuadable	Truly Unwilling
I don't want my kin to suffer more.	39	52
Others in my family would object.	30	34
Giving is complicated.	27	35
Doctors may not try to save my kin.	27	36
It's against my religion.	17	31
I don't want my relative disfigured.	13	45

Source: Adapted from Prottas and Batten, 1991b.

Persuading the Persuadable

The message content of public education ought to be determined by the concerns of the persuadable segment of the population so long as the 52 percent of people who are already willing are not alienated. The most important reason they give for refusal is based on a basic misapprehension—that an organ donor can suffer. In fact, organ donation procedures are performed only on the dead. This concern therefore seems to reflect a general fear that the medical system will treat the donor inappropriately if the family agrees to donate.

The postmortem nature of the donation may be a very difficult issue to address in a mass market context, but it implies that the core message of public education has to be changed. The message presently focuses on altruism and helping others, but the data indicate that much greater emphasis ought to be placed on reassuring the public that organ donation is considered only after all efforts at rescue have failed. This shifts the focus of the message from the good a donation does, which is not disputed or doubted by many, to the circumstances under which a donation is possible.

A second element that should be addressed is fear about the donation process itself. The concerns of the respondents, combined with what we know of their socioeconomic situation, implies that this persuadable group is not comfortable with or trustful of large medical or bureaucratic institutions. These people need to be assured that the donation process will not place confusing or embarrassing demands on them. Portraying the process as nonthreatening and simple would alleviate one of their biggest reservations. This can be done to a certain extent in the mass media, but it needs special emphasis when the family is actually contacted at the hospital.

The concern expressed that the donation process might be resisted by other family members and so engender conflict at a time of grief is the hardest to address. In all probability, it cannot be confronted directly. Perhaps the only way of dealing with it is to target other concerns and so decrease the likelihood that family conflict will exist.

Although blacks have the same concerns as whites, the importance of the concerns differs. With the exception of fear of prolonging suffering, persuadable blacks are far more worried about each issue than whites, particularly concerning the donation process itself and a general mistrust of doctors. Whereas both groups consider religion and disfigurement less important than other considerations, black respondents are nevertheless much more concerned about these matters than whites. Public education aimed at persuadable blacks therefore has to differ in several ways from that aimed at whites. The simplicity of the donation process requires more emphasis. The support of religious groups, especially churches with a large African-American membership, may also be important.

Is Public Education Worthwhile?

There is little reason to suppose that public education as presently practiced can make a significant contribution to increasing the supply of organs. More than half of the population is already effectively committed to donation; 20 percent appears to have decided against it. (It is possible that some members of this group could change their minds, but that would be a "point of sale" effect, not a marketing effect. The contact in the hospital is the "sales" step in organ donation.) At most, 29 percent of the population could be influenced by public education. No attempt to evaluate public education campaigns so far has been able to show that minds are changed or support is increased.

The Errors of Public Education: Whom to Persuade of What?

Millions of dollars are spent each year on public education, and little of it has any impact or even a coherent goal. Some efforts are based on inventive themes and slick presentations. Few show the least idea of whom they are trying to persuade of what.

The typical organ donation ad appears as a public service spot on local TV or radio. It emphasizes the need for transplantation or the moral worthiness of the act of donation. The medium conveying it is aimed at the buying public: young, white, and middle-class. As a result, the money is spent trying to convince the already converted of matters about which they have never expressed any doubt.

Most public education in support of organ donation violates every rule of effective marketing. There is no attempt to segment the market to discover who needs to be approached. There has been no attempt to understand the motivations of the public in order to tailor messages to meet the needs or allay the fears of donor families. Simply stated, most organ procurement organizations know nothing about marketing, and most marketing consultants know nothing about organ donation. Public education is therefore generally conceived by an alliance of the amateur and the ignorant.

Effective marketing requires careful market segmentation when the public sought is not homogeneous. And the American public is not homogeneous with regard to organ donation; both race and class matter a lot. Segmentation by these factors is therefore a simple and critical first step and has the advantage that these distinctions can be operationalized with relative ease. Residential patterns often segregate the public by both race and income, and print as well as broadcast media are available that are aimed at distinct populations, especially in large cities. If class distinctions are less easy to track than racial ones, there are still marketing channels designed to reach specific populations. Certain retailers and certain products find their primary markets among the working class and the less affluent, others among the more affluent.

In addition, American communities are rife with associations, institutions, clubs, fraternal organizations, and a variety of other grass-roots groupings. They may be more apparent in the suburbs than elsewhere, but they are nonetheless present in substantial numbers everywhere.

In general, public education programs have made no systematic attempts to target their efforts at the populations most in need of persuasion. Despite some minor attempts to approach the black community, no organization involved in organ transplants has systematically identified and accessed the media servicing the key communities where organ donation could reasonably be increased.

Equally important, there has been no effort to consider what message needs to be conveyed to any segment of the population or to consider the probability that any message will be accepted and acted on. Since the survey data indicate that a large part of the public is strongly committed to organ donation, generalized media exhortations are hardly necessary. Conversely, the segment of the public that seems unalterably opposed to organ donation will heed no plea. Only the segment in between, persuadable but with reservations, can profitably be addressed.

Then why is public education done at all? First, it allows medical professionals and even OPOs to deflect blame for inadequate donor supply. The implication is that lack of education among the public explains the problem. As the problem is actually professional noncooperation and the failure of the organ procurement system to overcome that resistance, this is a comforting proposition.

Second, public education is easy to do, visible, and alluring. A PR campaign is proof of activity. Nine out of ten people are convinced that they know how to mount such a campaign— all it requires is a catchy slogan, a heartrending photo, and money to buy space and time. It is also pretty much impossible to evaluate a public education effort negatively. If no donor increase occurs, other factors might account for the failure. At the very least, more time can be insisted on before the effort can be evaluated fairly. Indeed, some proponents of public education strongly advocate the need to start educational efforts among grade school children, thereby insuring themselves a generation or so before any evaluation is possible.

And these efforts are fun. They can be done in the comfort of an office. No hostile neurosurgeon treats you with contempt, and you don't have to show up in ICUs at inconvenient times or give in-service training to nurses in inaccessible hospitals. There is none of the frustration and failure that are inevitable when doing the more mundane and painful work of hospital development and cajoling medical professionals.

It is doubtful that any presently operational public education is worthwhile. First, only a very small percentage of the people hearing the message will have the misfortune of ever being in a situation of acting on it. Of that very small number, 70 percent are unlikely to have their views influenced—either because they already agree or because they are adamant in their opposition. On cost-efficiency grounds, public education has nothing to recommend it. Even on effectiveness grounds, it may be that improved "sales" are better suited to boosting donations than public education. More effective presentation of the donation alternative to a family after a potential donor has been identified has obvious advantages. It is directed at the audience that can donate, and it is interactive, allowing the particular concerns of that family to be addressed. In general, the point of marketing is to bring the consumer into the store; the sales force actually closes the deal. In organ donation, what brings a family into the store is an accident, followed by a referral from the hospital. The primary function of marketing is not applicable because it is the medical system, not the family, that decides if the family will be brought into contact with the transplant coordinator.

If public education is to make any contribution to organ supply, it can be but a modest one. The only way to improve its efficiency is to target it to the segments of the population that don't donate but might and to tailor the content of educational messages to the real concerns of those people. In effect, this requires targeting minority communities and working-class communities and assuring them that the organ procurement system is "user-friendly"—protective of the interests of the donor and of the family as a whole. Of course, it must also ensure that it is indeed protective of their rights. The irony is that the system is generally more responsive to families' concerns than the public messages it chooses to transmit indicate.

It must also not be forgotten that support for organ donation is lower among African-Americans and poorer Americans only in relative terms; the baseline of support is high in these communities too. The concerns of these communities also differ only in degree from those of other communities.

This indicates that targeting public education for organ donation can be done without compromising the ethical standards expected of the transplantation field. The messages sent reflect the reality of the organ procurement system; they are not misleading in any way. The communities concentrated on are not being asked to compromise strongly held values—the vast majority is supportive of organ donation or at least open to it.

Not only is targeting public education at the social and attitudinal segments of the American population where donation rates could be increased the most effective policy, but it is also a policy that can be pursued without apology.

Policies and Incentives

If public education can play only a secondary role in increasing organ supply, the question naturally arises whether alternatives to our present uncompensated voluntary system ought to be instituted. However, a change in procurement policies might increase the percentage of the total population willing to donate and so increase supply directly. In addition, it might indirectly lead to more families being asked. If the medical professions see a greater willingness to donate, they will be more likely to refer patients. (This possibility will be considered in Chapter Four.)

Several alternative policies have been considered by groups concerned with donor supply. One involves incentives to donor families. The buying and selling of organs is against the law in the United States, but the lure of the market is such that a variety of incentive proposals continue to be made. Other approaches have also been proposed, including tax credits and transplantation priority to families who have permitted donation.

The other major alternative involves altering some aspect of the permission process itself. Required request laws have been passed by both the federal government and a majority of states. Although they do not alter the rights of families, they do alter the donation process in that, in principle, all families will be asked. Presumed consent laws have not been enacted anywhere in the United States with regard to organ procurement but are law in several European nations. We have already called into question the efficacy of such laws; the issue now is their popularity.

Table 3.6 shows the public's levels of support for these various alternatives.

Table 3.6. Support for New Policies, by Attitude Group.

	Percentage of Respondents Expressing Strong Support		
Policy	Willing Donors	Persuadable Donors	Unwilling Donors
There should be national support for intensive public education.	44	31	14*
Donor families should get priority for transplantation.	27	18	17
Donor families should get tax credits.	14	7	8
Donor families should get cash payments.	9	8	5
Required request laws should be implemented.	25	17	7*
Presumed consent laws should be implemented.	7	2	3*

*Differences are statistically significant.
Source: Prottas and Batten, 1986b. Used by permission.

A survey by the National Kidney Foundation indicates that support for incentive policies among Americans has increased. Although it is hard to compare this survey to earlier ones, support for presumed consent laws and for payments to families seems to have grown—but neither reflects a majority view. The Foundation also found that the public is more supportive of incentives to donors that are somewhat indirect in character, such as payments to charities in individual names (National Kidney Foundation, 1992).

Across all groups, support for incentives systems is directly related to the indirect nature of the incentive offered. Priority to receive a transplant has consistently had broad support, and as an incentive, it is wholly symbolic. The chance that a family will have a member killed under circumstances making organ donation a possibility and then have a member in need of an organ transplant are vanishingly small. Beyond that, tax credits or charitable contributions are viewed more favorably than cash payments.

The data do not suggest that a policy change would increase the supply of donors. No new donors can be expected from the willing group, whose members are already willing to donate without compensation. Because willing donors outnumber those who might be motivated by incentives by more than two to one (52 percent versus 25 percent), incentive programs face a difficult challenge. Some people committed to the voluntary system will decline to donate if payments are introduced—surveys of donor families indicate this. To increase the supply of organs, incentive systems would have to alter the behavior of a very high percentage of nongivers while alienating very few people presently willing to give. At best, therefore, introducing the market into organ donation would not much increase the number of Americans willing to donate; at worst, it might decrease that number substantially. Of course, it would also drive the price of the system up as we would then be paying for what we are now getting free.

Overall, it is possible to say that the public is not very supportive of changes in the policies underlying our organ procurement system. The final answer seems to be that there is no pressing need to take steps to alter the public's role or place in organ donation. New policies have little support and might expose the system to large risks. Under these circumstances, more targeted public education efforts are the only defensible activities in this arena, and even they must be viewed as of marginal relevance to the total supply of organ donors.

Routine Retrieval: An Unconsidered Alternative

The commitment of the American public to the present organ procurement system renders most alternative systems impracticable at this time. However, routine retrieval proposals bypass the issue of public participation. No nation operates a system of involuntary organ donation, so its operational characteristics can only be imagined. In broad outline, such a system would be simple. When a potential donor died, all suitable organs would be removed for transplantation without consulting the family and without the family (or the deceased) having the right to refuse. Dispensations could be made for religious groups with fixed objections to the procedure, just as the military draft has procedures to deal with conscientious objectors.

Under such a system, neither the family nor the medical professionals treating the dying patient would have any discretion regarding the postmortem use of salvageable organs. It would still be necessary to identify potential donors, but since the social issue of family attitudes is avoided, various technical methods can be brought into play to facilitate donor identification. (Chapter Four discusses one such approach that can be implemented even under present policies.)

Routine retrieval has the clear potential for generating many more organ donors than we are likely to be able to find under any voluntary system. Such a policy, combined with routine information sharing between hospitals and organ procurement organizations, could easily lead to a three- or fourfold increase in the supply of transplantable organs. At present, only 25 to 30 percent of potential donors actually donate; in a nonvoluntary system, increasing that to 80 percent or more is conceivable.

There are certainly moral grounds for its adoption. The benefit that recipients receive from an organ transplant is obvious and requires no elucidation. With the exception of a small number of religious groups, there is agreement that the donor suffers no harm from the procurement procedure. (Very few Americans believe that being buried intact confers benefits in the afterlife.) The only ones who could suffer—psychologically, not physically—are the donors' families, and surveys show that only about 20 percent of them have categorical objections to donation. In contrast, the benefits to recipients are often life-saving and always life-enhancing in a major way.

There would be costs attached to routine retrieval—intangible ones whose magnitude is somewhat more difficult to estimate. The opportunity for altruism would be lost. Some observers argue that altruism has substantial social utility and that society ought to value systems that permit its exercise. However, the point of organ transplantation is to help people in need. It would be an odd inversion to structure the procurement system to foster altruism at the expense of saving lives. That might be likened to permitting poverty in order to allow charity to flourish.

But in a society that values individual freedom, coercion is itself a cost. In terms of rights denied, the cost does not seem high compared to the myriad of other rules enforced for the public good. Many states require people to wear seat belts while driving, and all states prohibit the use of certain classes of drugs because of their detrimental effects on the user. Denying a person the right to be buried with a healthy kidney hardly seems a very harsh or limiting imposition of state control. But in such matters, the views of third parties may not be the best test. If the public feels routine retrieval to be a harsh and unreasonable example of state coercion, it may be so. As no one has actually asked the public, we cannot know with certainty how such a policy would be regarded. However, based on the generally negative reaction to the much milder presumed consent alternative, it is safe to predict a strong negative response to routine retrieval.

As we shall see, medical professionals are even more committed to voluntarism than the general public. Routine retrieval would have to deal not only with public attitudes but with professionals' attitudes as well. As a practical matter, rejection by either group is sufficient to scuttle the policy.

Thus routine retrieval has no chance of becoming public policy in the immediate future, and any strong pressure from the transplantation community would do more harm than good by feeding public fears. Nevertheless, routine retrieval deserves more serious consideration than it has been given. Initially, this might have to be limited to academic observers and ethicists. Many scholars argue that routine retrieval is easily defensible on ethical grounds and that its rejection is indefensible. If such a consensus emerges, we may find ourselves, for the first time in a generation, with a real task for public education in the organ donation field.

4

Medical Professionals and Organ Procurement

THE PUBLIC IS WILLING to donate organs but must be given a chance. That chance is provided by certain medical professionals. Conversely, from the point of view of the organ procurement system, these professionals control access to potential donors and donor families. The medical teams that care for dying patients stand between the organ procurement system and the giving public, so the supply of organs depends on whether these intermediaries can be induced to play the role of liaison rather than that of obstacle.

In this chapter, we will consider exactly what doctors and nurses must do if organ procurement is to succeed, and we will discuss what is known about their willingness to do those tasks. In addition, we will address the operational and policy question of what can be done to increase their cooperation in organ procurement.

The Place of the Professional

It is impossible to overestimate the importance of staff cooperation, as the supply of organs is directly dependent on the level of cooperation obtained from doctors and nurses. This cooperation raises questions that are very different from those raised by family cooperation, but in its own way, it is just as difficult to obtain. A medical proefssional's initial role in organ

procurement is both the simplest and the most difficult: to identify potential donors in a timely fashion. This difficulty is not
technical, since any competent intensive care staff can anticipate which patients are terminal. But ICUs are very busy places,
and their staffs are dedicated to saving the lives of the critically
ill. It is both practically and psychologically difficult to take
the time to recognize an imminent failure and shift from concern for saving a life to concern for salvaging organs. If asked,
most ICU staff members could identify a suitable donor easily,
but the requirement is that they act spontaneously and proac-
tively. The result of such identification is a referral, notification of an organ procurement organization that a donor can
be found at a given ICU. This first step in the process is the
single most important factor in determining the supply of organs.

Following a referral, a physician, usually a neurosurgeon because of the nature of the injuries, must declare the donor brain-
dead. Brain death determination can be a time-consuming
process and in almost all cases serves no purpose except to permit organ removal.

Although brain death determination is merely a technical
step, informing the donor's family and explaining brain death
require complex social interaction. Families expect that the doctor will be the one to tell them of their relative's status, and
this applies to a declaration of death. Moreover, the concept
of brain death is not clearly understood by the public. It therefore falls to the physician to explain it to the grieving family.
Others—representatives of the OPO, nurses, clergy—may ask
permission for organ donation and further explain brain death,
but the declaring physician must introduce the subject and its
applicability to the patient.

The final responsibility of the ICU staff is donor maintenance. There is inevitably a period of time, from several hours to as much as a day, between brain death and organ removal. Patients must be stabilized, tests run, operating room time obtained, and surgical teams assembled. During this period, the cadaver remains in the ICU, and the staff must monitor its condition to ensure the viability of its organs and the continuation of its heartbeat (with machine support). This is a lengthy and, for some, emotionally difficult task. ICU staffs are dedicated to caring for the living, and this is monitoring the dead. Nor is this always easy. Once a person's brain is dead, the normal homeostatic processes of the body cease, so care is required to maintain fluid balances and look after other procurement-related matters.

The role of medical professionals in organ procurement is complex and demanding. Unlike families, medical professionals are not required to make a single, reactive decision in the midst of personal tragedy. Rather, they are expected to undertake a series of concrete, sequential activities, some technical or medical and others social and interactive. Their willingness to participate is therefore not a function of their support of organ donation per se but rather a function of their willingness to undertake a narrower series of responsibilities. These responsibilities may or may not be seen as integral to their primary functions, congruent with their personal beliefs, or reasonable with regard to the demands they make on time and emotional energy. In fact, professional support for organ procurement is probably best defined in terms of level of willingness to engage in the least attractive and least valued of these tasks.

Attitudes Compared

Just as the tasks of medical professionals vary, so do the professionals themselves. We have already alluded to the two most important groups, ICU nurses and neurophysicians (generally neurosurgeons). Other in-hospital professionals may play secondary but also important roles. The hospital CEO bears ultimate responsibility for organ procurement activities in the hospital, and CEO permission is a precondition for procurement. Lower in the hierarchy is the director of nursing (DON), who serves as both hospital administrator and senior nurse. Like the CEO, the DON's permission is a prerequisite for activity, and that support may be critical to the willingness of ICU nurses to cooperate. Each of these professionals has a different constellation of responsibilities regarding organ procurement, and each has a different, and in some cases conflicting, set of perceptions regarding the process and the role of medical professionals in it.

It is a commonplace among organ procurement specialists that nurses are the most and physicians the least supportive group in the hospital. A 1982 survey of the directors of the nation's largest OPOs reported that neurosurgeons were both the most important and least cooperative members of the hospital staff they had to deal with. Nurses were considered almost equally important but far more supportive (Prottas, 1983).

The attitudes of medical professionals has been quite consistent over time. The impressions of OPO directors in 1982 were validated four years later in the course of the only existing national survey of key medical professionals—the tables in this chapter are based on that survey. These data were in turn validated four years later by a detailed survey done in a large industrial state (Prottas and Batten, 1990). The levels of support and the reservations of doctors, nurses, and hospital administrators have shown remarkable stability.

On the face of it, there could hardly be a higher level of support among these professional groups for organ procurement. The personal attitudes of medical professionals are compared in Table 4.1. The responses of the general public to the same questions are provided for comparison. A vast majority approves of organ donation; it is an unambiguous cultural good. Nearly all medical professionals would consider donating their own organs. This level of support is not very different from that found in the social and racial groups from which these medical professionals come (they are overwhelmingly white and middle-class; neurosurgeons are also overwhelmingly male). The same observations apply to attitudes regarding willingness to donate the organs of a relative, although here medical professionals are far more supportive than other white middle-class respondents.

Most relevant professional groups are reasonably likely to communicate their feelings to their families. The only exception is neurosurgeons, who are not much more likely to have discussed this with their family than the general public.

Overall, the personal attitudes of medical professionals give no reason to anticipate the least difficulty in getting them to cooperate wholeheartedly in organ procurement, yet OPOs find it a continuous struggle to obtain the needed cooperation. Personal attitudes are clearly not the factors defining actual willingness to act.

Table 4.1. Personal Support.

Statement	Hospital Administrators	Directors of Nursing	Intensive Care Unit Nurses	Neurosurgeons	Public
Personally, I strongly approve of organ donation.	91	93	93	91	90
I would consider donating my own organs.	–	96	94	91	72
I would consider giving permission to have a family member's organs donated.	–	96	95	94	53
I have discussed my feelings about organ donation with my family.	–	68	71	52*	46

*Differences between professional groups are statistically significant.
Source: Adapted from Prottas and Batten, 1988.

Bottlenecks in the Process

Medical professionals may not act on their support of organ procurement for a number of reasons: they may have reservations about clinical aspects of the process, they may have concerns about interacting with the families of donors, or they may be unwilling to pay the time and emotional costs of involvement.

Clinical Issues

There are a number of areas where the technical concerns of medical professionals might influence their willingness to assist in organ procurement. To take the first step of making a referral, it is necessary to be aware of the criteria defining an organ donor. On the one hand, this is a matter not of attitude but of knowledge. More profoundly, however, it is an attitudinal issue. Organ donor criteria are not esoteric, and no trained nurse or physician could fail to learn and remember them with minimal effort. For these groups, knowledge is so easily obtained and so clear that not having it reflects not ignorance but indifference. As the responses to the first two statements in Table 4.2 show, both doctors and nurses believe that they do have the knowledge needed to identify donors. Nurses are more modest in their self-evaluation, but almost 70 percent believe that their colleagues know how to identify a potential donor. However, they disagree dramatically with physicians as to how well informed doctors are. Nurses see doctors as more ignorant than themselves. Physicians, in contrast, are virtually unanimous in their certainty of knowledge. In both their self-evaluation and their evaluation of physicians, the nurses are seconded by the other two groups surveyed.

85

Table 4.2. Clinical Issues.

Statement	Percentage of Respondents Agreeing			
	Hospital Administrators	Directors of Nursing	Intensive Care Unit Nurses	Neurosurgeons
Physicians are aware of the criteria that make a terminally ill patient a possible candidate for organ donation.	66*	55	49	96
Nurses are aware of the criteria that make a terminally ill patient a possible candidate for organ donation.	72	68	69	—
Medical and clinical guidelines for deciding if a patient is brain-dead are well established.	69*	56	53	88
Brain death criteria are generally accepted by the medical community.	83	60	62	91
Physicians don't like to become involved in making brain death decisions.	76*	87	81	44
I am comfortable designating a patient on a respirator as being a potential donor.	—	—	92	82
Medical protocols for treating a patient who may become an organ donor often conflict with procedures for protecting organs that may be transplanted.	—	48	58	59
Involvement of OPO staff in donor maintenance is appropriate.	—	—	—	60
Donor maintenance is appropriately part of a nurse's job.	—	—	92	—
Nurses are not resistant to caring for brain-dead cadavers.	—	—	72	—

*Differences between groups are statistically significant.
Source: Prottas and Batten, 1986a. Used by permission.

This reveals a theme. Neurosurgeons' self-perceptions differ from the perceptions of their co-workers. This is particularly surprising and problematical with regard to the ICU nurses. Professional cooperation in organ procurement requires their joint efforts. The physician's skills and legal rights make his or her cooperation necessary. Only the physician can declare death and permit access to the patient. But the nurse's role is also critical. Only the nurse knows the donor's family, and only the nurse's willingness to spend the time and effort necessary to maintain a donor can bring the process to a conclusion. Thus professional cooperation is essential, yet we find that nurses and neurosurgeons often differ profoundly in their evaluation of doctors' attitudes.

Neurophysicians are required to make the brain death determination, and they do not find that to be a technically controversial action. But even though 90 percent of neurosurgeons have no technical reservation about brain death, almost 45 percent believe that their colleagues don't like to make that determination! Nurses believe that 80 percent of doctors don't like to become involved in this process, and directors of nursing and hospital CEOs agree. This is a critical bottleneck in organ supply. Brain death determination is essential to organ procurement, yet in the view of 45 percent of neurosurgeons, their colleagues are uncomfortable being involved in the process. And this is considered by other staff to be a gross overestimation of their level of willingness. If the reason for these hesitations cannot be technical, we will have to look at other substantive concerns to identify its cause.

The cause does not appear to exist in the clinical sphere at all. Neurosurgeons express comfort regarding all clinical issues.

Neurosurgeons are confident that they can legitimately identify a respirator-dependent patient as a potential donor without compromising their medical responsibilities. The only area in which they do have reservations is instituting certain donor-related medical protocols. In general, the care of head injuries requires dehydrating a patient to counteract swelling. By contrast, maintaining a robust fluid volume is helpful in protecting the viability of organs. When such a conflict arises, medical ethics and organ procurement practices require, of course, that the patient be protected. In any case, this issue is irrelevant to the brain death question because no conflict in preferred protocols can arise after the patient is dead. Finally, we ought to note that nurses express great willingness to do the postmortem tasks required of them in an organ donation. Over 90 percent accept donor maintenance as a professional responsibility, and a smaller but still preponderant majority don't find caring for the cadaver a particularly emotional problem.

Interpersonal Issues

Although there are disagreements across groups as to how supportive physicians are, there appears to be no significant clinical reservation about organ procurement among these groups. The situation is quite different when we ask about family and interpersonal matters (see Table 4.3). Neurosurgeons accept the responsibility of explaining brain death to donor families, and the majority of them think that this is not a particularly difficult concept to explain. In this they differ from the other professionals involved. Fortunately, it is the neurosurgeons' accepted responsibility, so their views are the most pertinent. At the same time, over 40 percent of these physicians do consider it hard to explain brain death.

Table 4.3. Concerns of and About the Families of Donors.

Statement	Percentage of Respondents Agreeing			
	Hospital Administrators	Directors of Nursing	Intensive Care Unit Nurses	Neurosurgeons
It is the neurosurgeon's responsibility to explain brain death.	–	–	–	88
Brain death is hard to explain.	62*	65	67	41
Donor families would see a conflict for involved physicians to request organ donation.	–	–	–	48
Organ donation helps families grieve.	82*	86	79	66
My professional colleagues are somewhat reluctant to approach families about organ donation.	–	–	49	68*

*Differences are statistically significant.
Source: Adapted from Prottas and Batten, 1988.

This may partly explain why more than two-thirds of neurosurgeons believe that their colleagues are reluctant to approach families regarding organ donation. Here we have one of the most serious impediments to organ procurement in the medical system. If physicians are unwilling to approach families, it will adversely affect their willingness to initiate the process by identifying donors and undertaking brain death determination. This effect is potentially the most important, not the unwillingness to speak with families per se. Physicians don't have to speak with families about organ donation—a competent OPO representative can do that. Therefore, this reluctance on the part of physicians has important implications for the way OPOs must operate and the impact of public policies on organ supply. Both subjects will be examined shortly.

Concern about explaining brain death may be one aspect of the explanation of physician reluctance to approach donor families, but other factors also play a role. Almost half of neurosurgeons believe that families would see a conflict of interest if they raised the matter of organ donation. And even though two-thirds of neurosurgeons believe that organ donation helps a family, about 80 percent of all other professional groups think this way. More important, as shown in Chapter Three, the public has far more positive attitudes about donation and physician involvement than doctors attribute to them. Almost 80 percent of the public believes that organ donation helps a family deal with its grief, and only 20 percent feels that physician involvement in asking for organs could represent a conflict of interest.

Clearly, neurosurgeons have grave reservations about dealing with the families of potential donors. They are frightened by many aspects of the process and exaggerate these reservations. They do this despite the fact that most OPOs are diligent in conveying the readily available data on public support for donation and despite the fact that the professionals they work with have already assimilated this information. Only when dealing with technical or quasi-technical issues, such as brain death and its explanations, are doctors comfortable with the organ donation process.

Time and Emotional Costs

Having to deal with the families of donors is not the only demand that organ procurement makes on medical professionals. There are other costs of involvement—time, emotional wear and tear, legal exposure. There are also subjective factors that support and encourage cooperation.

All the involved medical professions find organ procurement emotionally demanding (see Table 4.4). As it usually involves the sudden death of a young healthy person, the bereavement of a family, and the failure of medical technologies to which they have dedicated their lives, this is hardly a startling finding. The impact of the time it takes to complete a donation is somewhat more surprising. Over 45 percent of neurosurgeons hesitate to become involved in donation because of the time demands. Admittedly, a brain death declaration can be time-consuming. Nurses see organ procurement as even more time-intensive, and in fact the time a nurse must commit is substantially more than that required of a physician.

Concern about legal liability is widespread among neurosurgeons but not among hospital administrators. The legal exposure of physicians in the field of organ donation is less than

Table 4.4. Subjective Costs of Involvement.

Statement	Percentage of Respondents Agreeing			
	Hospital Administrators	Directors of Nursing	Intensive Care Unit Nurses	Neurosurgeons
My professional colleagues find organ procurement emotionally demanding.	71*	70	84	74
Physicians are somewhat likely to hesitate to become involved in an organ donation because of the time involved.	—	—	—	46
Nurses find organ procurement activities somewhat time-consuming.	61	77	77	—
Hospital administrators find organ procurement activities somewhat time-consuming.	37	35	57	—
Physicians often express concern about their legal liability in the organ procurement process.	25*	40	30	51
Hospital administrators often express concern about the hospital's legal liability in the organ procurement process.	19	15	—	—
Clinicians feel that organ procurement activities are a professional responsibility.	—	—	75	51*

*Differences are statistically significant.
Source: Adapted from Prottas and Batten, 1988.

negligible. Hospital administrators, with their infamous sensitivity to legal risks, consider the matter trivial, yet half of the neurosurgeons surveyed believed that their colleagues were actively concerned!

Sources of Unwillingness

It is the interpersonal, not the technical, aspects of the process that daunt physicians (and to a lesser extent other professionals). Nurses as a group are more willing to act than physicians are primarily because they are less afraid of interacting with the families of donors. Nurses are less certain about the technical issues involved and have a stronger sense that brain death is a difficult idea to convey, but doctors are more reluctant to approach families and are more inclined to anticipate family hostility and resistance. This "fleeing without pursuit"—for families are supportive and cooperative—even shows up in their baseless fears of legal liability.

But if neurosurgeons are more suspicious of involvement in organ procurement than nurses are, neither group is monolithic. If public policy and OPO practice are to increase willingness to cooperate, the differences among doctors and nurses may be as important as the differences between them.

Differences Among Physicians

Several factors tend to distinguish more supportive from less supportive physicians: older doctors are less intimidated by donor families than younger ones, physicians are influenced by the kinds of hospitals they practice in and by whether they have had actual experience with organ donation, and most important, neurosurgeons' attitudes are affected by their own definition of their professional role.

Neurosurgeons practicing in teaching hospitals and in hospitals with large ICUs were found to be less affected by many of the concerns typical of their professional peers (Prottas and Batten, 1986a). They see less likelihood of legal complications and more benefit to the family of the chance to donate. They also believe that their colleagues are more willing to make brain death decisions than surgeons who did not work in teaching hospitals or who work in smaller ICUs. Finally, the time costs were less likely to dissuade them from cooperation. The effects of having already been involved in an organ donation were similar to those of hospital affiliation and ICU size: by most measures, physicians who have participated in a donation are more supportive than those who have not.

Being in a teaching hospital presumably exposes physicians to broader medical concerns than those emerging from their clinical practice. They are in contact with other specialists and are perhaps more aware of the benefits that new medical technologies, including transplantation, can confer on patients other than their own. In the same way, physicians whose practice brings them into frequent contact with potential donors may find the issues of organ procurement more familiar and hence less threatening. Finally, actual experience with a donation may help demystify the process and increase support.

Although organ procurement can be a difficult experience, it is not likely to be as hard as physicians imagine. Families are more supportive than doctors believe, and OPOs make strenuous efforts to minimize the burden on surgeons. Indeed, each of these environmental factors may act to increase support by reassuring a doctor that involvement in organ procurement is not terra incognita but part of a well-understood and appreciated medical system.

Each of the factors mentioned has a positive effect, but the attitude of professional peers and the perception of professional legitimation have by far the greatest influence on neurosurgeons' attitudes. A neurosurgeon who believes that identifying donors, declaring brain death, and dealing with the family are part of the responsibilities of the profession is far more supportive and cooperative. All identified impediments, family contacts, time, costs, and other factors are seen as less daunting. Undertaking difficult tasks as part of his or her calling is experienced quite differently from doing so in support of a desirable but professionally irrelevant social good.

Nurse Cooperation

Intensive care unit nurses follow a similar pattern, but one that differs in interesting ways. Like neurosurgeons, ICU nurses are strongly affected by their perception of their professional responsibilities. Unlike physicians, however, this is not the most important factor influencing them. Whereas donation experience has only a small impact on doctors, it has the greatest single impact on ICU nurses. The donation experience, with all of its emotional and time demands, is so positive and satisfying for nurses that they are generally very willing to repeat it. Finally, we have also found that nurses are influenced by doctors. Nurses who see doctors as more supportive are themselves more supportive and willing to cooperate (Prottas and Batten, 1986a).

Motivating Cooperation: The Politics of Professional Education

Professional education has been a mainstay of OPOs for years. There are psychological and practical justifications for the terminology but very little substantive justification. Professional education is more exhortation than education. The goal is not to inform so much as to mobilize. Few ICU nurses and fewer doctors really need to be told much in the way of technical or medical facts regarding organ donation. All they need to know is that an OPO exists and what it will do; beyond that, they need to be reminded of the necessity for organ procurement. Salience and not information is the "right true end" of professional education. Calling it education does have attractions—indeed, irresistible ones. First, in most medical contexts, education is good by definition. Second, for the primary target of professional education—nurses—education is a requirement. In most states, nurses must take a certain number of hours of continuing education to maintain their license. Hospitals have an interest in facilitating this process, and a couple of hours of professional education on organ procurement serves everyone nicely.

Virtually every OPO in the country spends a large part of its time on professional education in one form or another. In fact, the average organ procurement specialist spends more time on professional education than on organ procurement. This is not the best strategy. Nurses are already more supportive than physicians, and though nurses' attitudes are affected by physicians' attitudes, this effect is not reciprocal. Targeting physicians would be more cost-effective both because they are the narrowest point in the pipeline and because they can increase the level of cooperation of others. The major arguments against targeting doctors is that they will not come to the educational meetings and that they will not listen to the OPO staff doing the educating. It is the experience of most OPOs that one-on-one exhortations, conducted with deference, may be helpful, but no other forum will attract or influence doctors.

By contrast, nurses can be *sent* to organ donation meetings, have professional reasons to attend them (continuing education credits), and often have an interest in coming in any case. They are also willing to learn, especially since many organ procurement specialists are nurses themselves.

The 35 percent of OPO time that officially goes toward professional education is, of course, an underestimation of the total effort that is being expended on these tasks (Prottas, 1983). An organ procurement is itself an effective piece of professional education—at least for nurses. Most OPOs are very sensitive to this fact and will, on occasion, actually go through with a procurement they know will not yield a usable organ simply to educate new hospital staff. In addition, all OPOs make it a practice to provide feedback to all professionals involved in a donation with a view to thanking them and maintaining their goodwill. It would not be an exaggeration to say that half of all the efforts of an OPO are dedicated to motivating medical professionals.

Changing Moral Basis of Professional Involvement

The need for this prodigious expenditure of effort essentially follows from the application of the principles of voluntarism and altruism to medical cooperation in organ procurement.

Until the passage of required request and routine inquiry laws, medical professionals were treated according to the same principles as donor families regarding their participation in organ procurement. This meant that the assumption was that professional cooperation was both necessary and a matter of *personal* moral beliefs.

This was a striking combination of assumptions. The practical

97

necessity of medical cooperation has been discussed and is ir-reducible in present circumstances. The ethical necessity for voluntary involvement is less obvious and appears to rest on the belief that physicians have a right to control who will have access to their patients and, by extension in this context, to the families of their patients. This attitude seems to be an out-growth of the control a physician has over the care a patient receives, as no one but the responsible physician may prescribe for or treat a patient without the physician's permission, and no one may intervene regarding the physical fate of the patient, even postmortem, without the physician's consent. It has been the universal policy of OPOs not to examine patient records, discuss patient suitability with nurses, or approach families with-out the explicit permission of the attending physician.

The necessity for physician permission has been tied to the free right of physicians to deny that right of access. The ground of the right to deny has traditionally been founded on consider-ations analogous to the right of a family to refuse an organ do-nation request—that is, a person's cooperation in organ dona-tion is a personal, ethical decision that must be uncoerced. Yet the validity of this analogy has been called into question. Why is physician cooperation in organ donation essentially personal or ethical? Must cooperation be voluntary and spontaneous in the same way that family cooperation ought to be? And if med-ical cooperation is not analogous to family cooperation, what policy interventions can legitimately be applied?

Alternative Policies: Incentives

True to our culture and history, the first answers to these ques-tions revolved around money. If medical cooperation was not in the ethical sphere, perhaps it was in the market sphere. This approach was very ill received in the organ procurement community, on two grounds. First, that community remained committed to the personal, ethical model of medical cooperation, and second, it was skeptical of the efficacy of such incentives, even if their inappropriateness was overlooked.

At least on the empirical matter, these instincts were sound. Neither nurses nor physicians support the introduction of marketlike incentives into the organ donation field. They agree that monetary payments to the key parties is not a policy alternative. Both nurses and doctors find the idea of paying families unacceptable, and both reject the idea of medical professionals being paid to support organ donation. Interestingly, each professional more strongly rejects receiving payment itself than it rejects payment for the other (see Table 4.5).

Alternative Policies: Public Intervention

This rejection of market incentives does not extend nearly so strongly to other public interventions in the donation process. Medical professionals are not universally hostile to other forms of public policy interventions. As Table 4.6 shows, there is substantial medical support for two key public interventions: brain death legislation and required request laws. Nurses are almost unanimous in supporting legislation defining brain death, and even a majority of neurosurgeons support such a step. This is striking given the strong hostility of the medical profession to any lay intervention into medical practice, decision making, or criteria. Almost as striking are attitudes toward the passage of required request legislation.

The putative goal of this legislation is to remove the right

Table 4.5. Attitudes Toward Recommendations for Compensation of Professionals or Family Members.

Statement	Percentage of Respondents Agreeing			
	Hospital Administrators	Directors of Nursing	Intensive Care Unit Nurses	Neurosurgeons
Physicians should receive a fee for evaluating potential donors whether the donation takes place or not.	47	36	22	18
Nursing staff should receive extra financial compensation for participating in organ procurement activities.	6	8	13	21
The government should provide cash incentives for families of brain-dead potential donors who grant their consent.	9	10	13	10
Tax credits should be provided to families of brain-dead potential donors.	26	32	40	25
Priority to receive an organ transplant should be given as an incentive for families of brain-dead patients who grant their consent.	40	42	49	—

Source: Prottas and Batten, 1986a. Used by permission.

Table 4.6. Attitudes Toward Legislation.

Statement	Percentage of Respondents Agreeing			
	Hospital Administrators	Directors of Nursing	Intensive Care Unit Nurses	Neurosurgeons
A law should be passed that defines brain death.	–	84	91	59
A law should be passed that presumes consent for organ donation for all brain-dead patients.	11	11	12	12
Hospitals should be required to participate in organ donation efforts.	25	38	62	39

Source: Prottas and Batten, 1986a. Used by permission.

of medical players to control access to the families of potential organ donors. As this diminishes the autonomy of medical professionals involved in the process, a negative reaction could be anticipated, and in fact only nurses express majority support for the innovation. However, a very respectable minority of neurosurgeons is also supportive—almost 40 percent.

It may be that the supportive neurosurgeons see required request laws as a way of diminishing their fear of interaction with donor families. If the request is routine and mandatory, they may feel insulated from the emotional burden of confronting the family.

However, it is also possible that the structure of required request laws has minimized physician concern. These laws demand not that the clinician become involved but that the hospital develop protocols. Clinicians may therefore see these regulations as moving the burden of involvement from them to the hospital administration. The attitude of hospital administrators suggests that this is their perception; only 25 percent favor required request laws, the lowest level of support found among any group.

Emerging Moral Assumptions: Public Values

Recent years have witnessed a remarkable increase in public involvement in organ procurement. One major thread of that involvement has been external intervention into the relationship between the physician and the organ donor and family. The speed at which this has occurred is impressive. By and large, the medical community has not resisted this intervention, either as professionals or as individuals. This raises two questions. First, why do doctors, nurses, and other medical professionals not object to public intervention in this relationship? Second, why do we need to be concerned with their views and preferences now that the public has defined their responsibilities and removed the voluntary nature of their involvement?

More than half of neurosurgeons support a legal definition of death, and some 40 percent support a legal requirement that families of potential donors be approached regarding donation. Both these steps socialize a previously private relationship and substitute policy for professional judgment. Organ procurement is one of the very few areas where medical professionals have been willing to surrender those prerogatives. As we shall see, the medical component is no less routinizable in organ distribution than in organ procurement, but there the profession has resisted public control systematically, with fair unanimity and success.

Two factors have made this relative openness to socialization possible (recognize that it is only a relative openness—a bare majority of neurosurgeons support brain death legislation, and only a minority support required request laws). These factors are families and death. Physicians are afraid of the families of donors, dread the personal encounter with them, anticipate hostility, imagine charges of unprofessional conduct, and fear legal action. At the same time, almost all physicians involved believe in organ transplantation and donation—they consider both laudable activities. The former is professionally sanctioned and efficacious, and the latter is morally praiseworthy. A dilemma therefore emerges between an honest desire to support a worthwhile activity and a strong disinclination to engage in the key tasks necessary to do so. For physicians, brain death laws and required request laws can provide at least a partial resolution of the conflict. Laws defining brain death are almost wholly symbolic, but for physicians, it is a protective symbolism. Brain death laws validate and excuse the painful step of declaring a person dead who might appear to be alive—a brain-dead cadaver is still warm and breathing. At the same time, these laws provide physicians with assurance that their legal position is protected and that no serious legal attack can be mounted against them. In this way, these laws may be supported because they reduce the fear of involvement and allow medical professionals to support a morally and professionally approved activity.

Required request laws have similar attractions. Symbolically, they validate the request process—indeed, they characterize it as a right of families. They define the responsibility as an organizational one, and although physicians may find their particular responsibilities unchanged, the hospital accepts the overall duty to arrange the process. In this way, physicians may act under the color of another authority. For those who want to assist in organ donation on moral and social grounds, being able to approach the process as a legal obligation, an organizationally assigned task, and as a duty to patient families can certainly diminish the perceived likelihood of interpersonal conflict.

Finally, the sine qua non of professional willingness to acquiesce is death. Although traditionally the donation process was defined as part of the physician-patient relationship, it was always a bit anomalous because the patient no longer lived. Thus organ donation came under the physician-patient rubric by extension or momentum. No outside intervention was legitimate between a living patient and the doctor, but once the patient was dead, a host of other considerations might come into play. This fact helps explain the surprising willingness of professionals to countenance public involvement in donation issues and at the same time defines the limits of the practical implications of that intervention—for required request laws do not end the key role of medical professionals in organ donation.

Required Request Laws

Limits of Required Request

The central limitations of required request laws as coercive measures have to do with the interpenetration of the postmortem donation process with the premortem treatment and evaluation process. In reality, the donation process cannot start only after the patient is dead. Death must be anticipated. Optimally, this allows the beginning of certain testing procedures involving the patient's histocompatibility and identifying the presence of certain diseases, notably hepatitis and AIDS. Plans for a brain death declaration must be put into effect before death, as must plans to maintain the donor while permissions are obtained and logistics are worked out. Due to time restraints, a request for organ donation made without preparation at the time of death cannot be effectively acted on. Hence intrusion into the premortem domain of the physician is required and depends wholly on the physician's sufferance.

Equally important is dependence on the physician's expertise. No legal reform can alter the fact that only a very small proportion of dying patients are suitable organ donors. Identifying them requires the proactive exercise of professional knowledge. Whereas required request laws insist on justification if a family was not approached, there can be no serious challenge to a physician's clinical judgment that a patient was not suitable on medical grounds. The dependence of the process on the clinical expertise of physicians is at least partly, and perhaps largely, a matter of access rather than technical judgment. In some cases, to be sure, only a trained physician could say if a donor is medically suitable or if the proper treatment of a moribund patient is compatible with maintenance of the organs in a usable state. However, in most cases, technical judgment is secondary to the fact that no decisions can be made about a living patient except by the treating physician.

Before death has been officially declared by a physician, no patient can be examined or evaluated without the doctor's permission. In a sense, no relevant information exists about the patient except that provided by the treating physician or a consulting physician. Technical details on temperature, blood electrolytes, and the like are merely data; the patient's state is socially identical with a physician's evaluation of those data. This monopoly on patient access and treatment is the universally approved right of the medical profession. Although it clearly protects the medical profession in a number of ways, its most persuasive foundation is that it protects the patient by ensuring that only medical considerations are allowed to play a role in treatment. However, its effect on organ donation is to ensure that no legal changes enacted can diminish the dominance of the medical profession in the organ donation process. Organ procurement is predicated on a potential donor's physical state, and even in technically obvious situations, only a physician may make an authoritative social and legal determination of that state. Medical professionals are inherently the gatekeepers of organ procurement.

106

Uses of Required Request

The policy implications are several, and the futility of required request laws is not one of them. Required request laws do not and cannot end the voluntary nature of medical involvement in organ procurement, but they can alter some of the key terms of professional education. First, these laws can give an active OPO both access to hospitals and a service to perform for hospitals. All hospitals participating in Medicare must have an organ procurement protocol and a designated person for approaching families. OPOs can provide both an acceptable system and trained personnel. Just as OPOs can provide continuing education credits to nurses and so be in a position to offer something as well as asking for help, now they can help a hospital fulfill its obligations under required request laws.

To a lesser degree, required request laws have also added a song to the OPOs' repertoire in dealing with physicians—although here the effect is certainly less. Insofar as the hospital has expectations that doctors will consistently identify organ donors, the OPO can now help them fulfill their responsibility to the hospital. Insofar as doctors now have to enter into the medical record the reason why they did not initiate an organ donation request, the cost of not cooperating has increased. Active and aggressive OPOs use this in their approaches to doctors—now not only can they work at making cooperation as easy as possible, but they can also argue that noncooperation has work and time implications.

In the final analysis, public intervention in the professional roles in organ procurement has been primarily symbolic. As a

107

practical matter, it has been impossible to coerce cooperation. The professional's role remains proactive, and even under optimum circumstances, proactive behavior is difficult to enforce. Nor are the circumstances of organ donation anything like optimal. There are innumerable medical reasons—or excuses—for not designating a patient a suitable donor, and none can be gainsaid except by another physician. Socially, it is easy to render inoperative any requirement for approaching a family for permission to procure organs: it only requires that the request be poorly expressed or ambiguously presented or even insensitively worded to get a rejection. Hostility is not required; indifference will suffice. In such intimate matters, law is far too crude a tool to be used. And as we have seen, required request laws are not really meant to be used in this way—they are aimed at protocols and practices; at hospitals, not clinicians; and they are by and large without penalty. They state a social expectation, not a positive requirement of law.

But as social expectations they are important. First, they not only state an expectation but also reflect one—one shared by the medical profession and the public. Organ donation is praiseworthy; an imprimatur of authoritative action by government doesn't make it so, but it does reinforce, publicize, and legitimize it. And the various forms of public involvement are important not only for what they reiterate but also for the new proposition they present. These laws define a new right to oppose a professional prerogative. The right posited is that of the public to act altruistically when an objective possibility to do so exists. Families, say Congress and state legislatures, have a right to be asked. This right imposes an obligation on people in a position to initiate the asking process. And this obligation overwhelms their personal right not to be involved and their professional right to decide how to deal with their patients' needs. This right can be asserted only because of the special circumstances of organ donation and brain death. It cannot be effectively enforced against the monopoly of information held by medical professionals, but it has been asserted, and this represents a significant change in the terms of debate regarding the role of the public and of professionals in organ procurement.

A new right has been validated. In the process of organ transplantation, the donation itself is on the boundary of the medical system. Public involvement in the transplant itself is not a prospect; public involvement in the distribution system, though growing, is still weak and without a strong philosophical defense. But the donation itself clearly touches on matters of a sensitive and nonprofessional nature. It is, in effect, both the beginning of the transplantation and the primary point at which the medical world touches the social. And so it is reasonable that this is the place where the public would be the most willing to act to assert nonprofessional values and impose social expectations. So even if the socialization of organ donation is symbolic, it is powerfully so. Not only does it assert a social right, but it invents that right and declares its superiority to the competing and hitherto dominant values of professional autonomy.

New Policy: Extending Required Request

Required request laws are not the only or even the logical end of the development of diminished professional autonomy in organ procurement. The principle of required request laws is that cooperation with organ procurement efforts is not a matter of choice for the medical profession. The practice of required request laws is that they affirm this principle without taking any steps to implement it. Medical discretion in organ procurement is essentially a function of control over information. Only the doctors and nurses in the ICU have timely information on the status of potential donors. Required request laws tell them that they ought to use that information only to ensure that families are approached. But the reasons that these professionals do not choose to cooperate in procurement efforts are not changed by required request laws. Therefore, there is no very persuasive reason to believe that their behavior will be much altered. Indeed, there is no indication that required request laws have changed behavior markedly.

The challenge for policy makers is to find ways to make the principle that medical professionals ought not exercise discretion in organ procurement into a practical policy that excludes them, as far as possible, from exercising what is now defined as illegitimate discretion. This discretion is based on control over information. If that control is diminished, discretion is diminished proportionately. A policy of routine referral would do this (Prottas, 1988). Under such a policy, the organ procurement system would be routinely informed when a potential donor was admitted to a hospital. It would then be the responsibility of the OPO to contact the ICU treating that patient to determine status and suitability. This step would substitute for the present referral from the ICU itself. If the potential donor were suitable, the process could proceed as it now does. If the donor were not suitable, due to recovery or medical contraindications, the process would end. If the prognosis were still uncertain, contact would be reinitiated later.

The primary advantage of routine referral would be to eliminate the bottleneck at the hospital that presently constrains the supply of organs. The present system is essentially perverse: it requires medical professionals to take a proactive role and relegates the procurement system to a reactive one. But the procurement system is the responsible party regarding organ donation. It has no other responsibility and so has both the motivation and the resources to take an active role. ICU staffs, by contrast, have other primary and pressing duties. Requiring that they take the initiative and responsibility is analogous to procuring organs only if the family initiated the procurement process. That would simplify the procedure, but no serious system of organ procurement could be founded on such behavior. Yet our procurement system is currently dependent on just such self-initiated actions by disinterested third parties in the hospital ICU.

Admittedly, routine referral does have some problems. It would be necessary to define which hospital admissions are reported to the OPO. This is a technical problem, and its resolution would depend on whether the problem of missed admissions was more serious than that of fruitless and inappropriate calls from the OPO. The process of informing the OPO would not necessarily even require human involvement. Granting the OPO limited access to the hospital's information system might allow a computer-to-computer exchange. At worst, the process would require a small time commitment from clerical personnel at the hospital.

The social problems might prove somewhat more intractable. With OPOs calling the hospital, they risk being perceived as "vultures," eagerly awaiting death. At least some of the calls will be inappropriate. This may not be a serious problem for nurses. As we have seen, nurses are very supportive of organ donation, and routine referral will both increase the number of donations they are involved in and decrease the responsibility they bear. It would be irrelevant for doctors, who rarely interact with the OPO directly on referrals in any case. The OPO staff will probably be the ones who find it most difficult to accommodate this death-detecting role because it highlights a basic but unpalatable fact of their profession. The OPOs *are* on the lookout for deaths—organ procurement depends on death and tragedy. But awaiting a death is not the same as wishing for one, and in any case, the psychological problems of OPO staff ought not define organ procurement policy. These problems are inherently more manageable than those of professional education because they occur within the OPO system rather than in a separate system that OPOs seek to manipulate.

Routine referral would not solve all of the problems with professional cooperation. Nurses and doctors could still refuse to cooperate based on the kinds of considerations we have already discussed. Nor would this policy allow the OPO to bypass the medical professionals and go directly to families. But it would make noncooperation much less likely, in that failure to act is far easier to justify than an overt refusal to do so.

At present, only about a third of potential donors are referred to OPOs. Routine referral would not have to be extraordinarily successful for it to identify more donors than this. Even if criteria were excessively strict and medical staff more resistant than they are likely to be, required referral would certainly increase the number of families approached about donation. In addition, it would give reality to the principle of family primacy embodied in required request laws and reduce our expectations of medical professionals to more fair and reasonable levels. Finally, its demands on hospitals would be no greater, and perhaps less arduous, than those imposed by any serious attempt to adhere to required request laws. Its only negative aspect may be that it forces the parties to the organ procurement process to face their own place in it. Medical professionals would have to admit that society has stripped them of a prerogative that they have long had, even if they have never shown many signs of enjoying it. OPOs would have to admit that they are waiting for death and that it is tragedy that makes their work possible. But if American families can see through tragedy to the needs of others, it doesn't seem too much to ask the other key players to face realities in the same cause.

5

The Ethics and Politics of Distribution

THE "GIFT OF LIFE" can only be made through an organ procurement organization. Unless the gift can then be delivered to a recipient, the process has failed—an undelivered gift is no gift at all. The delivery of organs to needy individuals is the responsibility of the organ-sharing system; the ethical and operational characteristics of that system are the subject of this chapter.

No aspect of the organ transplantation system is so essentially political as organ sharing. Organ donation has to do with families and kindness and organ procurement with the retrieval of a usable resource, but organ distribution has to do with *who gets what*, and that is a zero-sum game. The supply of organs is fixed in the short run; the demand inevitably exceeds the supply, and so the organ distribution system determines who will and will not be left in want. Ultimately the want refers to patients, but proximally it refers to surgeons. The operation of the organ-sharing system therefore touches the practice of each of the nation's transplant surgeons very directly, determining both the quantity and the characteristics of the resources they need in their work.

The Way It Has Almost Always Been

Nowhere has the American genius for individual initiative and local action been more successful or more distressing than in the field of organ procurement. "Every surgeon a king, and every city a kingdom" has been the rule. The Uniform Anatomical Gift Act, the basic legal underpinning of organ procurement, states that the recipient of the gift of the organ is the retrieving physician. Unfortunately, this legal formalism has often been taken quite literally by transplant surgeons operating OPOs.

Traditional System

The local power base of organ procurement has been responsible for the system's excellent success in locating and obtaining donors; it has also been the deciding factor in how these organs are allocated among patients in need. Most OPOs were created to provide a single transplant surgeon and team with needed organs. The OPO was staffed by nurses employed by the hospital housing the team and operated under the immediate direction of the transplant surgeon. These agencies served as medical supply units, making organ distribution simple and unproblematical. All procured organs were used locally—if the surgeon wanted them. All medical criteria regarding recipient suitability were set by the transplant surgeon.

As late as 1987, this was the way most OPOs operated. The only other models were the OPOs that served more than one transplant hospital. In these cases, where more formal and explicit organ-sharing rules had to be developed, the dominance of local surgeons was even more visible. When transplant teams from several hospitals joined together to direct an organ procurement organization, the first issue discussed was how the organs would be distributed. Two answers predominated: the geographical approach and the turn-taking approach.

In geographically based allocations, each transplant hospital is allocated certain community hospitals from which only it could draw organs. (The allocated hospitals were usually not consulted. The allocation was based on relationships, variously and unilaterally defined, that predated the formation of the OPO.) All organs obtained in affiliated hospitals were treated as if they had been donated at the transplant hospital. Turf conflicts would often develop when the scale of one hospital's transplant program failed to keep pace with the productivity of its stable of community hospitals. Regular attempts were then made by "have-nots" to reallocate community hospitals.

The turn-taking system generally avoided this problem. Under it, each transplant hospital team takes turns being on call as the excision team. If a team does not wish to use a given organ, the next hospital on the list is called. In both of these systems, the key factor is that a transplant team has first refusal on organs procured. The organs are essentially allocated to the surgical teams and not the transplant patients. This generally meant that if two kidneys were obtained, the surgeon was free to transplant at least one of them into any patient on his or her list; the second had to be shared according to agreed-on criteria. These criteria varied by OPO, but even in the most progressive systems, they included both hospital-related and patient-specific criteria.

The central characteristics of organ allocation in the traditional system were, first, that the hospital and not the patient was the primary unit to which the allocation was made and, second, that the criteria by which allocation decisions were made were always local and often informal and unwritten. This is not to say that these allocation decisions were necessarily objectionable. In all cases, the core ethical considerations were deeply embedded in the central ethics of the medical profession.

That is, the procuring transplant surgeon had control of a scarce and valuable commodity and acted on the obligation to look after the best interests of *his or her patients*. The right and ability to do so were enhanced by a very strange phenomenon—the persistent disagreement among medical professionals as to what factors define the best interests of the recipient of a transplant.

With every transplant surgeon insisting that his or her allocation criteria were superior to all others, the dispute persisted even as the organ procurement system was transferring many organs among transplant centers. There simply weren't many agreed-on rules. In the period from 1980 to 1984, almost half of all kidney transplants were done with an organ imported from a distant procurement center (Prottas, 1984). Because surgeons' standards differed, this figure varied greatly from area to area. San Francisco, the largest transplant center in the world, neither imported nor exported organs, while Philadelphia, with one of the largest organ procurement organizations in the world, exported 80 percent of its kidneys. But for the system as a whole, organ sharing was an essential part of the transplantation process.

The operation of this huge sharing system reflected a curious mix of science and arbitrary choices. On the science side was the computer registry of the United Network for Organ Sharing (UNOS). This registry was accessible by every OPO in the nation and listed (in principle) every person awaiting a kidney in the United States, along with their human leukocyte antigen (HLA) characteristics, sensitivity, time on the waiting list, and the OPO listing them. This computerized system could provide any OPO with a list of all potential recipients who were theoretically well suited, in immunological terms, to receive each available kidney. However, each OPO was at liberty to use this information as it wished; the system was purely informational and contained no standardized criteria for organ sharing. In practice, ad hoc rules and "old boy" networks distributed America's organs.

When an OPO had an organ it could not place locally, the standard procedure was to access the UNOS computer to find other suitable recipients, matched first by the number of HLA antigens they shared with the donor organ. Another factor that came into play in the choice of an OPO was the presence of backup recipients. As all organs have only limited cold ischemic time, it is very desirable that the importing OPO have several possible recipients so that if cross-matching shows one to be positive and therefore incompatible, there is a chance that another can receive the organ with minimal delay. In effect, this means that OPOs with large lists are preferred; it is therefore better to be waiting for a kidney transplant in Boston than in Wichita.

Because time matters, OPOs also gave preference to nearby OPOs. If a close-by center could not use the organ, there might still be time to reexport it to a third location. Friendships counted as well, since trust is important on both sides of an interagency exchange. The importing agency has to have faith not only in the veracity of the exporting OPO but also in its skills: Was the organ removed skillfully? Has it been properly maintained? Is the donor information exact? and so on. OPOs that supplied organs that were not as represented or caused difficulties in the past found it impossible to export. Similarly, OPOs that could not be trusted to act quickly and place an organ tended to be excluded from the organ-sharing system.

And finally, there was reciprocity. As the system was highly discretionary, placing organs with OPOs that had many to export was clearly a preferred practice. Old boy networks were the norm, even though a complex medical and computer system was employed to operate it.

Norms and Criteria: Efficiency and Equity

Between 1982 and 1992, more than eighty thousand kidneys were transplanted in the United States and an equal number abroad. Kidney transplantation is such a large business and has been going on for so long that an impressive data set has been accumulated on outcomes, patient characteristics, organ characteristics, and related matters. Such data are valuable for resolving the key questions that arise in kidney distribution: the preferred level of HLA matching (tissue compatibility) between donor and recipient and the impact of cold ischemic time (the period during which a kidney is cooled and without a blood supply).

These are central issues; they relate to the question of how to maximize the probability of transplant success. If tissue matching has a large impact on graft survival, finding a well-matched recipient among the twenty-three thousand people awaiting a kidney is important. This suggests a national search and the frequent sharing of organs. If cold ischemic time has a large impact on graft survival, speed in locating a donor is important, and this suggests a smaller, more circumscribed search and infrequent organ sharing. If organ viability is strongly affected by preservation time, the logistics of organ sharing may be as important as the science of tissue matching. With tens of thousands of cases available for analysis, the transplant community could be expected to resolve these issues with a fair degree of scientific rigor. That it has failed to do so is one of the mysteries of medical science—or medical sociology.

The old boy sharing system did take cognizance of these issues, even if it didn't explicitly or systematically include them. Medical efficacy has always been the central language of its public discourse. The meaning of *efficacy* is quite close to that of *efficiency* in the language of economists. This means that the basic test applied to allocation rules is whether they result in placing organs into patients with the highest probability of graft survival. The entire dispute around HLA matching and preservation times is couched in these terms.

Proponents and opponents of matching as the preeminent sharing criterion differ on the kinds of evidence in which they place their faith. Matching advocates refer to the works of Paul Terasaki in America and Gerhard Opelz in Germany on large data sets (Cook and Terasaki, 1988; Opelz, 1988, 1991). These men employ statistical analysis to predict transplant outcomes using the combined data from hundreds of transplant centers. Their results are unambiguous: HLA matching improves transplant outcomes, and the effect increases over time—that is, the difference in survival rates of well-matched and poorly matched transplants is greater at five years than at one year. Using the same type of analysis, Opelz also finds that preservation times up to forty hours have no effect on outcomes. These data are not new, and in Europe they have long been the basis of organ-sharing practices (Lowy, forthcoming). In America, however, only a minority of surgeons accept it. Most American surgeons object to the pooling of data from different transplant centers and insist that the experience of individual centers does not support Terasaki and Opelz or at least that doubt remains (Salvatierra, 1988).

At the beginning of the cyclosporine era, the doubters gained increased influence because they argued that the new drug rendered the old data irrelevant, and, of course, new data did not exist. (In the early and mid 1980s, cyclosporine became the drug of choice for immunosuppression. It was found to be more effective than previous treatment options, and it acted in a somewhat different biochemical manner. Its introduction called into question the relevance of previous data on transplant outcomes.) Organ sharing dropped radically, and matching was used less. However, by 1988, the debate had returned to its old form, with the same arguments being repeated by the same people. By 1988, sufficient data had been gathered on cyclosporine transplants for statistical analysis to show that the old relationshps were unchanged. Also unchanged was the rejection of the analysis.

At one level, the conflict is between the scientific and the clinical world view. The findings of large-scale data analysis differ in kind from what a clinician considers critical information. Transplant surgeons are, in general, more clinicians than scientists. They are acutely aware of the differences among individuals, and for them each patient is unique. Their experience is that graft survival is the result of a more complex series of factors than just HLA matching. The statistical idea of isolating an effect by holding other factors constant generates answers often inconsistent with the experience and working reality of clinical practitioners. Such people deal with one complex patient at a time, and no patient's characteristics can be "held constant."

Complicating the debate are the political implications of different answers in the debate over matching and ischemic time. In the extreme instance—when HLA matching matters and ischemic time doesn't—organ allocation can be reduced to a universal algorithm. At the margin, there can be disputes over whether or not small differences in match matter, but the core of the allocation decision will be objective and quantitative. In this case, control over organ donation moves both professionally and geographically—professionally from surgeons to biomedical researchers, geographically from local to central decision making.

The HLA system is very complex; mapping, techniques for testing, the relationship between various antigens, and the impact of some antigens in relationship to others all make it a very specialized field. This is the realm of the biochemist and the biostatistician, and some of the active and respected practitioners in the field are not physicians at all. If HLA matching is to determine organ allocation, surgeons will have to surrender control over decisions that affect them and their patients to professionals they cannot evaluate and to criteria whose impact they cannot accurately anticipate. Their resistance to doing so is comprehensible. In addition, the locus of allocation decisions would change from local medical communities to a centralized organization.

On practical grounds, any dependence on HLA matching as an allocation tool requires universal cooperation. Many physicians involved in transplantation are convinced of the efficacy of matching, and many OPOs allocate their organs at least in part on matching criteria. However, their commitment to matching could hurt their own transplant programs over time because while they would share organs for better-matched patients, other OPOs would not reciprocate. The result would be a net outflow of organs. So it is impossible, as a practical matter, to use HLA matching for organ allocation across OPOs unless all transplant programs are operating under the same rules. Failing that, a moral Gresham's law pertains: the determination to keep one's organs drives out the willingness to share for better results. As we shall see, part of the pressure to inaugurate a national agency overseeing organ allocation came from transplant programs committed to HLA matching and unable to afford to pursue that goal independently.

If HLA matching is not as important as short preservation times, locally based clinicians should retain more control over organ usage. Many physicians believe that except in the case of perfectly matched organs, HLA matching is only a minor factor in graft survival. The predominant factors are clinical and reflect the same complexity of decision criteria common to most medical treatments. Within accepted practice standards, therefore, the allocation of organs is, in this view, better done locally, where cold ischemic time can be minimized. Organs should be shared only when, in the judgment of the responsible physicians, no local recipient is suitable.

One additional argument has been presented against any system of HLA-driven national organ sharing, and that is the incentive argument. Organ procurement is a time-consuming and often emotionally draining task, and doctors and nurses, it is argued, would be less willing to engage in it if the organs procured were to go elsewhere. This is the case made in support of various forms of local priority for locally procured organs. Insofar as the argument is applied to medical personnel in community hospitals, it consists of unsupported assertion. Insofar as it is meant to apply to OPO employees, it is incorrect. But as a description of the surgeons' own willingness to pursue organ procurement, it must be taken seriously.

Transplant surgeons are key players in the organ procurement process, if only because they actually excise the organs. This is a task that often has to be done at inconvenient times and in distant places. If a physician says that a doctor will be less willing to do this if the procured organ is to be allocated to another's patient, this becomes a significant argument.

Pressures for Change

Government Readiness

Despite the general desire on the part of transplant clinicians to be allowed to pursue organ procurement and allocation in their own way, pressures began to grow in the early 1980s for new standardized rules and new players. These pressures resulted in a substantial socialization of organ procurement and allocation and consequently in substantial changes. The terms of debate and the people at the table changed as a result of a series of factors, including the increased scale of the transplant industry, the multiplication of payers and costs, media (and political) manipulations, and differences within the transplant community itself.

The growth of the transplant industry itself was a major factor. Between 1982 and 1992, the number of transplants performed in the United States tripled, and the number of transplant centers increased even more dramatically. There are now almost eight hundred transplant programs, involving some 270 hospitals, in the United States (United Network for Organ Sharing, 1992). In 1990, organ procurement was a $200 million business.

Much of this money came directly from the federal government via its support for the renal transplantation program. Even though the Reagan and Bush administrations argued that the government had no need to involve itself in transplantation, the fact was that it was already paying for over 80 percent of all transplant costs. (The figure has now dropped to perhaps 65 percent as the number of privately funded nonrenal transplants has increased.) Almost as important, these payments were the best investment in the federal portfolio. It has long been understood, at least by Congress and the professionals in the executive branch, that a kidney transplant saved the ESRD program money because the alternative was maintaining a Medicare beneficiary on dialysis. A transplant not only eliminated dialysis costs but, after a grace period, removed many patients from Medicare coverage entirely. What was only slowly being realized was that the cumulative effects of an ongoing transplant program might actually be saving sizable amounts of money, even by federal standards (Eggers, 1984).

By 1985, more than nineteen thousand Americans were walking around with a transplanted kidney (Eggers, 1988). The increased scale of the renal transplant program and the improved success rates of the procedure may have swelled that number to well over thirty-five thousand by 1992. The cost of the dialysis program was therefore substantially reduced by the success of the transplant program. The federal government thus found itself paying for a financially and, as we shall see, politically significant program. This realization increased the government's desire to play a more active role in organ transplantation policy. It prepared the ground for what followed.

Transplant Community

Significant segments of the transplantation community also had reasons to support federal involvement. While renal transplantation was growing at a steady 8 to 10 percent a year, nonrenal transplantation was also becoming an important activity. Heart and liver transplantation was burgeoning; in 1991, 2,100 hearts and 3,000 livers were transplanted (United Network for Organ Sharing, 1992). The number of hospitals performing these procedures increased even more markedly. But in 1984, when the increases were just beginning, the medical professionals committed to them saw the need for government legitimation. This legitimation, though largely symbolic, was important and had both a positive and a negative aspect. On the one hand, the transplant community wanted formal recognition that heart and liver transplants were clinically efficacious activities and not just experimental procedures. On the other hand, they needed to escape the taint of the ESRD program.

All Medicaid programs and many private insurers look to the Medicare program for direction regarding what procedures ought to be covered. So long as Medicare considers a procedure experimental, other payers have a reason and an excuse for refusing to pay for it. Doctors and hospitals involved in heart and liver transplantation therefore had good reason for wanting the federal government to declare their work clinically efficacious and to begin to cover it under Medicare.

There were several obstacles to this step, none of them scientific. In clinical terms, by 1984 the outcomes of heart and liver transplantation were perfectly comparable to those of kidney transplantation. In scientific terms, there was no justification for the experimental designation. In financial terms, there was very little risk to the federal government in recognizing heart and liver transplantation as a legitimate medical procedure. Liver transplantation is a treatment suitable to two general groups of conditions. It can be used to replace the nonfunctioning liver of infants suffering from an inherited liver malfunction, most often biliary atresia; the age and life expectancy of these infants essentially excludes them from being covered by federal health insurance. The other group of potential liver recipients consists of young adults with liver failure due to various causes. They would be eligible for Medicare only if they had been disabled by another cause prior to suffering liver failure, a very rare circumstance.

So the strong pressure from liver transplant surgeons to get Medicare to cover liver transplants was not motivated by the desire to obtain large amounts of Medicare money but by the desire to have the federal government validate their procedure and so encourage other payers to provide coverage. In 1984, after a National Institutes of Health Consensus Conference, they triumphed, in a modest way. Medicare rules were changed that year so that the Medicare system would pay for liver transplants in children. As no children with the suitable illnesses were or could be eligible for Medicare, this decision had a charmingly Catch-22 air. The federal government agreed to pay for liver transplantation on the understanding that it would not have to do so. Nevertheless, the liver transplantation community had gone to the federal government for help and obtained it.

The heart transplant community did not find it so easy. The

ESRD trauma touched heart transplants more closely than livers. By most standards, the ESRD program had been successful. It was intended to provide universal access to an expensive life-saving technology, thereby avoiding the "God committees" of the early 1970s. The program was completely successful in this. Moreover, the per-unit cost of the program was actually decreasing in real terms since its inauguration, even during a decade of very high inflation in other medical costs. The problem is that the ESRD program was many times the size Congress was led to expect when it passed the enabling legislation. Congress enacted the ESRD program expecting it to serve seventeen thousand people in its first years and grow to a maximum of perhaps thirty-five thousand at some unspecified time in the future. These data came from the nephrology community, based on estimates of the incidence of renal failure in the nation. In 1991, more than 140,000 patients were being treated under the program at a cost of about $4 billion, and Congress had been traumatized (Health Care Financing Administration, 1992).

Although the applicability of this experience to heart transplantation was nil, media estimates of the demand for heart replacements—running to tens of thousands of procedures a year—made the administration and Congress very resistant to permitting Medicare to cover heart transplants. They imagined a second ESRD program.

By 1984, it was clear that somehow they had become utterly convinced of their nightmare. In 1982, the Health Care Financing Administration (HCFA) had authorized a national study to estimate the Medicare implications of covering heart transplants; that study was completed by 1984. Running to fifteen hundred pages, the *National Heart Transplantation Study*, reported by Roger Evans and colleagues, found that the cost of covering heart transplants under the Medicare system was trivial. Pointing out that organ supply limitations would hold the total number of heart transplants under two thousand a year for the foreseeable future, the study found that at most two hundred or so of those transplants would be done on Medicare-eligible patients. The impact on the $100 billion–plus Medicare budget would be infinitesimally small. However, the administration refused to release the study. As its findings were common knowledge in the transplant community, concerned parties began to search for allies to free the report. The National Task Force on Organ Transplantation was persuaded to request formally that the heart study be released, stating that it was needed for the completion of the group's work. These and other pressures ultimately forced the study's publication and with it the development of a new Medicare policy on heart transplantation.

Under the new rules, Medicare would cover this procedure in selected hospitals. As in the case of liver transplantation, the implication of the decision for other payers was of more importance than the direct impact on federal money. But for the organ procurement and transplantation system, the most important effect was that another segment of the medical community had socialized the transplantation system. In insisting on obtaining Medicare coverage, these physicians and hospitals had called for the aid of Congress, certain groups in the administration, and the National Task Force, itself a publicly appointed body. Heart and liver transplant surgeons, by entering the public arena and mobilizing allies to further their interests, were admitting that organ procurement and allocation policies were not solely within the purview of the medical profession. The very terms of debate they used undermined the traditional system. The task force and Congress were urged to act to further goals of access and equity. Arguments were made regarding cost efficiency, the relative value of different standard medical treatments, the cost of caring for terminal patients versus the cost of replacing their organs, even the societal advantages of returning young adults to the work force. The price of federal legitimation was public involvement, and both the heart and liver transplant communities were willing to pay the price—although they probably did not fully recognize the longer-range implications.

Even segments of the kidney transplantation community wanted changes badly enough to seek allies beyond the medical community. One such segment has already been alluded to—believers in organ sharing by HLA criteria who felt that they were being taken advantage of by others who would not share on that basis. But another factor was also at work. For the first time since the passage of the ESRD program, money was becoming a factor in kidney transplantation. Cyclosporine had made heart and liver transplantation possible, and it had also increased the one-year graft survival of kidney transplantation from 55 percent to 85 percent. By 1984, its use was absolutely standard and, most physicians would argue, medically required. Alternative therapies without cyclosporine had become or were becoming bad practice. The problem was that cyclosporine is ten times as expensive as earlier drugs. Traditional immunosuppressive therapy might cost $700 a year; therapy using cyclosporine might run to $7,000, and under Medicare rules, outpatient drugs were not covered.

Ability to pay was once again a significant issue in kidney transplantation. This was a matter of concern within the transplantation community. Many people found this distressing on general grounds of equity, and physicians were concerned that their patients were being denied access to care. Finally, most surgeons objected on professional grounds to the overlay of financial issues onto clinical decisions and saw such an overlay as counterproductive. Patients on cyclosporine did so much better than those not receiving it that doctors argued that cyclosporine actually decreased total posttransplant costs by reducing hospital stays.

The combination of these arguments induced Congress to charge the National Task Force with producing a report on immunosuppressive drug coverage separately and prior to its final report. The expectation of Congress was clear—it was asking for a mechanism for payment. Once the task force began meeting, arguments from the medical community were presented to a very sympathetic audience. The *Report on Immunosuppressive Therapies* (National Task Force on Organ Transplantation, 1985) strongly supported payments for immunosuppressive outpatient drugs, and more than a year prior to the passage of the 1988 Catastrophic Care Act, these particular drugs were being provided at government expense to transplant recipients. For the third time, money and technology had brought the transplant community to the government asking for help, and for the third time, help was forthcoming.

Public Players

The federal government had been the sole support of the transplant community since 1972, but neither the community nor the government had taken much notice of this fact. As long as the situation was stable, both parties pretended they had nothing to do with each other. The organ procurement system, 100 percent dependent on ESRD money, was virtually ignored by the source of its financing, and the organ procurement system in turn resented any interference from outside, which was in any case minimal. As late as 1983, nonrenal transplantation was a minor and unusual procedure, and kidney transplantation was a federal monopsony. But growth and change forced certain parts of the transplant profession to the attention of the government. Legitimation was needed for nonrenal transplantation, money was needed for new drugs, and from the point of view of parts of the transplant community, assistance was needed to deal with increased scale.

Probably none of the groups who approached HCFA and Congress quite understood the implications of their actions. They expected that they could get what they needed and be left alone to operate the system unsupervised, just as before. Based on the experience of the ESRD system, which made transplantation possible in the first place, this was a reasonable expectation. Two factors seem to have upset this calculation: first, the need to include nonmedical personnel in the decision making and, second, the political and media appeal of the subject. The argument made to Congress, HCFA, and the Task Force had to be structured in broad, nonclinical terms. Pleas for medical coverage of immunosuppressive drugs appealed to the initial access goals of the ESRD program, to the different social and especially racial impact of the cost of drugs, and to rather complex economic analyses. Professional government economists aimed to show that the direct costs of cyclosporine did not in fact add to the cost of transplantation because its use led to improved outcomes and decreased complications. In none of these arguments did physicians have a special status. Unwittingly, the medical professional had undermined its monopoly over transplantation policy in order to obtain some immediate benefits.

By itself this might not have been enough to alter the arena of decision making in transplantation, but other factors were making public involvement attractive or necessary from other points of view. Organ transplantation makes good copy and provides opportunities for a public figure to get onto a "motherhood" issue. In 1991, a dozen stories on the topic appeared in the *New York Times* and almost as many in the *Washington Post*, the *Chicago Tribune*, the *Boston Globe*, and the *Atlanta Constitution*. *USA Today* actually ran sixteen articles. Earlier a man named Charley Fiske had set the stage for the "save a child" motif in his attempt to get a liver transplant to save his daughter's life. Liver transplantation proved an almost perfect subject for media coverage. The technology was new and dramatic, the costs were high, and the patients were young children. Feature stories in newspapers, TV specials, and heartfelt pleas by desperate families became almost commonplace.

The issue was irresistible to politicians as well. President Reagan could not resist adding his own voice to the pleas for donors, even though the administration position was that organ transplantation was not the business of the government. In Congress, no hearing that touched on transplantation was complete without testimony from a recent recipient or the mother of a child in need. Perhaps without intending to exploit patients and their families, the media attention and the public pleas did raise a legitimate governmental concern: was the organ procurement and transplantation system operating effectively and equitably? The public and political perception was that it was seriously flawed.

Considering the way the issue was presented, this conclusion was inevitable. A shortage of organs is the basic reality of organ transplantation; the first questions politicians ask are why and how can this be fixed? The first round of answers enraged the transplant community by suggesting that paying for organs would increase the supply. Congress rejected this solution; in 1984, the National Organ Transplantation Act made it illegal to buy or sell human organs. This step was widely supported by the transplant community and others—it affirmed the moral underpinning of the present system, but it left unresolved the question of how to improve it. By this time, certain key members of Congress, notably Representative Henry Waxman of California and Senator Albert Gore of Tennessee, were committed to the proposition that something had to be done. In partial agreement were members of the Reagan administration, committed to the proposition that something had to be done—but not by them.

Congress felt that it had to deal with organ-sharing practices as well as with the question of organ supply. Equity in organ distribution was seen as important both as a value in itself and because it might have implications for the public's attitude toward donation, which is sensitive to the perceived justice of the sharing system. When a series of articles in the *Pittsburgh Press* (Schneider and Flaherty, 1985) charged that wealthy foreign nationals were being given priority access to transplantable organs, the result was a decrease in the donation rate of the

Pittsburgh-based OPO. Congress therefore saw several reasons to act aggressively in the organ procurement and sharing field.

Even as the transplantation community sought to involve the government, it nonetheless remained suspicious of Congress and its motives and offended by the assumption that the system needed fixing. The community was ambivalent and divided: some members were determined to keep the federal government at arm's length, while others were looking to the government to help solve their problems.

The Republican administrations were fairly consistent in their opposition to increased government involvement but operated under some crippling disadvantages. They could not deny that a problem existed, if for no other reason than that President Reagan had acknowledged that it did and made national pleas for help. They could insist that "private efforts" ought to solve the problem, but insofar as that implied simply waiting for someone else to do something, it was not an acceptable strategy for Republican members of Congress. They did not want to oppose legislation that called for more organs and their fair distribution. Finally, there was the matter of the ESRD program, which at the time was paying for 80 percent of all transplant costs. Clearly, it was too late to insist that organ transplantation was not a matter of legitimate federal concern.

For these reasons, the administration could not effectively fight the National Organ Transplantation Act of 1984. What it could do is delay the implementation of that act pending the report of its appointed task force. This accelerated the change in the nature of organ sharing in the United States.

The New System Takes Shape

The central player in the present system is the Organ Procurement and Transplantation Network (OPTN). This organization, under a contract with the Division of Transplantation in the Public Health Service, is responsible for setting standards and rules regarding the distribution of all human organs procured in the United States. It also has the responsibility of certifying all organ procurement organizations and transplantation hospitals for membership in the organization. OPTN membership is required for reimbursement under the ESRD program, and for hospitals doing transplants, is a condition for reimbursement under the Medicare system. In 1984, the contract to operate the OPTN was given to the United Network for Organ Sharing, which had until then been a subdivision of the Southeast Organ Procurement Foundation (SEOPF), a voluntary association of transplant hospitals and OPOs that provided assistance in organ sharing to its members and, through a computerized recipient listing system (the UNOS system), played a central role in kidney distribution nationwide. It was structured and operated on the model of a professional association. Its board consisted solely of transplant professionals, and it depended on an extensive committee structure to provide leadership and direction. At the time, there was no real alternative to UNOS as a contractee. However, after the passage of the National Organ Transplantation Act in 1984, the operating style and power of UNOS was radically transformed.

The OPTN took its initial shape as the result of the interaction of congressional expectations and the National Task Force's own agenda. Congress expected that each of the requirements of the National Organ Transplantation Act would be implemented simultaneously; however, administration-imposed delays meant that it came about in stages. The result was that the final form of the OPTN emerged from an additive process; the provisions of the 1984 act were added to the recommendation of the task force, and then the transplant-related provisions of the 1986 Omnibus Reconciliation Act were added.

This process is most clearly reflected in the final requirements the government imposed on the governance structure of the OPTN and on its powers over the organ procurement and distribution system. The 1984 act specified a fairly wide representation of interests on the OPTN's board, including patients and representatives of public and voluntary health associations in addition to transplant surgeons. However, it did not specify the allocation of seats, the exact role of the board, or any other concrete operational issue. Its directions set a broad standard for comprehensive representation without imposing a particular form of governance.

The task force extended the governance requirements further (National Task Force on Organ Transplantation, 1986). As part of its recommendation that the Department of Health and Human Services certify all OPOs, it proposed that the governance standards be applied to all OPOs as a condition for certification. These standards required majority representation of non–transplant surgeons on OPO boards of directors. In addition, it urged that the governing board of the OPTN be structured in the same way. UNOS resisted these mandates, so that the first time it applied for the OPTN contract, it was rejected, largely on the grounds that its plan effectively excluded nonmedical representation. In its second attempt to obtain the OPTN contract,

UNOS formally acquiesced to federal requirements. Operationally, the change was not as great as formerly; however, the granting of the OPTN contract in 1986 marked a watershed in the politics of organ sharing. Not only was there, for the first time, a national organization with control over the use of human organs, but its board of directors contained only a minority of transplant surgeons. Organ sharing was explicitly placed under the control of people not directly involved in the process.

This shift of power to a national and broadly representative body was all the more critical because it was seconded by a very substantial delegation of power to the OPTN. In its original conception, and even in the Task Force report, the OPTN was seen as a voluntary organization, although any transplant hospital or OPO that wanted to share organs through the OPTN had to be a member of it. This would have made it difficult—but not impossible—to remain independent: in 1984, the largest kidney transplant center in the nation neither exported nor imported organs. However, when Congress enacted many of the Task Force's recommendations in 1986, it went much further. Membership in the OPTN was required for certification of an OPO, and no hospital with a transplant program could receive Medicare funds unless it was a member.

The OPTN was no longer a voluntary organization. About 270 hospitals in the United States perform organ transplants, including all of the largest teaching institutions in the major medical centers. None of these could function without joining the OPTN. They could not, under the Omnibus Budget Reconciliation Act of 1986, even have the option of forgoing Medicare reimbursement for the transplants they do because the law requires a cutoff of *all* Medicare payments. Membership in the

OPTN is now a prerequisite for operating any organ transplantation program, whether paid for by public funds or not.

In effect, the membership committee of the OPTN is the gatekeeper for institutions wanting to enter the transplantation community. Heretofore, no quasi-private organization had this power, and even the government itself could not control entry into this industry. In theory, the government could refuse to pay for a transplant done at a noncertified hospital, but it could not stop a hospital from doing a transplant paid for from other sources. Since 100 percent of liver and 90 percent of heart transplants are funded by other payers, the federal government had only partial control over the transplant industry. The OPTN had complete control. It also had complete control over the procurement industry, as membership in the OPTN was required for certification as an organ procurement organization.

Between 1983 and 1986, the organ-sharing system of the United States had gone from being a semiformal, voluntary information-sharing system to being the arbiter of organ procurement, distribution, and use for the entire nation. In 1983, the United States had an organ procurement system of exceptional local strength and negligible national presence. There were no equivalents to the European models of Scandia Transplant, Eurotransplant, or the French and British national systems, all of which operated under imposed rules of sharing. By 1986, the comparison with European systems had been turned completely on its head. The power of the OPTN exceeded them all. It controlled access to every aspect of the system, from procurement to transplantation, and it had the right to set any rules it wished regarding distribution. But the OPTN did not want to exercise these rights.

How Organ Sharing Operates

Although the structure of the OPTN represented a break from the past, the actual operation of the organization exhibited considerable continuity. The professional staff of the new organization simply transferred from UNOS's parent organization, the Southeast Organ Procurement Foundation. With them came the SEOPF's operating style—the style of a professional association in which deference to the professional members and emphasis on consensus and nonintervention are central. UNOS/ SEOPF had not initially been supportive of a national organ-sharing agency. When it became clear that such an agency would be founded (and funded), the group still tended to see it in a conservative light, as a new organization changing as little as possible from the existing system. It therefore urged less public and more medical and professional representation and more local and less national power. Though overruled by the government on both matters, the new organization nonetheless retained a minimalist approach to its rights and responsibilities.

This disinclination to exercise its mandated power has taken many forms. The OPTN was required to develop a unified system of rules for the sharing of organs. These rules did not have to extend to the way organs were shared among patients within an OPO but were meant to define the criteria for interagency sharing. In fact, a number of specific rules were actually written into the National Task Force report, leading to the development of a point system (based on HLA, waiting time, sensitivity, and logistical factors) to identify which patient should be offered any given organ. It is a mandatory system intended to impose consistency on the way shared organs are to be used. Inevitably, many OPOs and transplant centers objected to the point system on one ground or another. The OPTN's response was to open an escape hatch, allowing any OPO to submit its own sharing system for approval. If approved, that OPO would be allowed to apply its own standards. Many have done so (United Network for Organ Sharing, 1989a). In effect, the OPTN declared that the national rules are to be treated as a "default," to apply only to the centers that don't prefer another system. At the outset, the exceptions were invited to swallow up the rule.

That OPOs are required to have explicit rules for organ sharing is a considerable step toward nationalization of the system, but the fact that each can substitute its own rules for the OPTN criteria means that it is still sorely fragmented. The OPTN was unwilling to impose on professional colleagues even where required to do so. Even more striking is that the response to disagreement was not to seek a national-level compromise, binding on all and satisfactory to most, but rather to revert to the traditional model of local dominance.

The OPTN rules for nonrenal sharing reflect a different but analogous pattern. Whereas a majority of kidneys are transplanted locally, the majority of nonrenal organs are transplanted outside the area in which they are procured. The rules for sharing are therefore very important to nonrenal transplant centers and had been developed by the largest centers even prior to the OPTN's founding. However, they were developed for a system very different from the one now in place. They were structured for a small system dominated by a small number of large transplant centers. The present system contains almost eight hundred transplant programs, in more than 270 hospitals.

There is broad agreement that the present sharing rules for nonrenal transplants are seriously flawed. In particular, the growth of heart and liver waiting lists makes the rules giving priority to the very sickest patients wasteful; a desperately ill patient has a smaller chance of doing well with a transplant than a patient in an earlier stage of illness. Similarly, current rules facilitate retransplantation, even though a person who has rejected one liver is more likely to reject the second. Many medical professionals are unhappy about these rules, but the OPTN has been hesitant to revise them as it would involve interference at the local level and possible conflict with professional colleagues.

This unwillingness to challenge local dominance extended to rejection of the explicit desires of Congress. The issue of nonresident aliens and their access to organs became a matter of public concern in 1984. (Nonresident aliens are defined as non-Americans who do not live in the United States. Noncitizen residents ought, by general agreement, to be treated like all other residents.) After much discussion, the National Task Force on Organ Transplantation recommended a quota, limiting the number of kidneys that could be transplanted into nonresident aliens, and agreed that nonrenal transplants into foreign nationals should not be done at all. In 1986, the inspector general of the Department of Health and Human Services (HHS) issued a report on the issue of nonresident aliens, arguing that it was a serious problem that was diverting organs and funding from the ESRD program. Congress agreed, and pursuant to the recommendations, it was decided that nonresidents ought to be treated differently with regard to access to transplantable organs ("New HCFA Rules May . . . ," 1987).

The OPTN looked into this matter with a committee of its

143

own and came to a quite different conclusion. It asserted that the issue of nonresident aliens had been "exaggerated in the media" and concluded that "there is no present need for restrictive policies with regard to the transplantation of non-resident aliens" and that therefore "transplantation of non-resident aliens shall in general only be done in transplant centers with well-established, historical patterns of international referral and reputation" in the area of renal care (United Network for Organ Sharing, 1988).

Not only were the recommendations and directives of Congress and the task force rejected, but the status quo in regard to nonresident aliens was reinforced. The only policy adopted by UNOS was further to limit nonresident transplants to centers already performing them. This step contradicted the premise that no problem actually existed.

The juxtaposition of the two positions reflects parallel forces within the organization. The general rejection of outside involvement in the allocation rules reflects UNOS's determination to maintain the independence of the medical profession in organ-sharing decisions. The recommendation that these transplants be limited to centers already doing them reflects deference to strong local forces.

This tendency to treat transplantation as an industry to be protected has brought UNOS into direct conflict with the primary actor on the federal government's side, the Health Care Financing Administration. Although the OPTN was unwilling to interfere in local affairs in most instances, it had taken a stronger tack regarding the certification of nonrenal transplant centers. Both UNOS and the HCFA have criteria for determining the acceptability of transplant programs. In many aspects, these criteria coincide, and some HCFA criteria are more stringent than those of UNOS. However, in one particular requirement, UNOS imposed tougher rules than the HCFA: UNOS criteria require that the physicians involved in a transplant program meet certain training standards. The HCFA has no such rule. UNOS criteria led to rejection of a heart transplant program application for OPTN membership. Without such membership, the program faced closure. The hospital appealed to the HCFA, which forced UNOS to grant provisional membership.

The HCFA's intervention was not based on a desire for greater public oversight of the procurement and transplantation system but rather on its belief that UNOS, as a provider organization, was acting to keep other providers from entering the industry. This specific conflict over a single heart transplant center was resolved by negotiation, but it led to far broader intervention by the HCFA in organ distribution.

In the course of this dispute, HHS realized that membership in UNOS was a precondition for receiving Medicare funds, which also meant that UNOS came under the scrutiny of the public agency charged with administering the Medicare program. HHS concluded that the powers granted to the OPTN were government powers requiring government oversight. In particular, UNOS could not use its power to exclude potential competitors from entering the transplantation business. This realization led to a modification of the OPTN's contract in February 1988. The new contract gave the secretary of HHS the right to review all membership requirements and to cancel the OPTN's contract if UNOS adopted any membership policy that, in the secretary's judgment, adversely affects Medicare or

Medicaid patients, is not scientifically supported, or is not in the "public interest" (United Network for Organ Sharing, 1988).

The HHS decision applied to membership policies and was designed to prevent restraint of trade. However, the decision seemed to validate the principle that the public grant of power to the OPTN permitted and perhaps even required direct public oversight of OPTN decisions. After all, it was argued, many UNOS policies had a more direct impact on Medicare and Medicaid patients and the public interest than membership criteria did. During the summer of 1988, pressure within HHS increased for more comprehensive and more direct public oversight of OPTN policies and practices. By July, this had taken the form of the Interagency Coordinating Committee (ICC) with broad powers over OPTN policy-making. This committee, made up entirely of government representatives, could examine all UNOS policies and "provide advice on any contract modifications," including forcing UNOS to change its policies or face cancellation of its OPTN contract.

The ICC has extended the Medicare-UNOS membership argument to justify direct oversight of all UNOS policies. Because adherence to UNOS's policies is a condition of membership and membership is a condition of Medicare reimbursement, the HCFA argued that the ICC must approve all UNOS policies. UNOS and the transplant community reacted with great concern. To quote a special edition of its newsletter: "UNOS feels it would be an unwise and improper step if such a committee were, in effect, to assume hands-on control over the development of standards and membership criteria. It is important for all transplant professionals, patients, families, interested individuals and related organizations, associations and advocacy groups to be aware of the formation of this committee . . . and to realize its potential for significantly altering policies formulated, agreed upon and adopted by the transplant community with broad input from the aforementioned groups" (United Network for Organ Sharing, 1988).

Final say on organ-sharing policy has effectively been removed from the transplant community and vested in a government unit. In 1989, HHS formally decided that it would have final power over OPTN rules and that pending its decisions, the OPTN could not enforce its policies (United Network for Organ Sharing, 1989b). In 1984, the United States had no decision-making unit above the local level in organ distribution, and even its regional coordination agencies were purely voluntary. Only a minority of agencies had any written policies regarding organ sharing, and where such policies existed, they did so solely at the pleasure of transplant surgeons directing the procurement agencies. In 1990, the issue became how closely the federal government would monitor a national-level organization that set mandatory organ-sharing policies for the nation.

Indeed, the entire discussion of who ought to make organ allocation decisions has undergone a revolutionary shift. The federal government is considering proposals that would require that all OPOs adhere to a single, uniform principle in organ allocation. This plan would require that all OPOs allocate organs from a single list and that regional and institutional variations among the OPOs play no role in the allocation system. Only a minority of the OPOs that serve multiple transplant centers currently operate in this way. In fact, it was only with reluctance that some federal policy makers dropped the idea that there ought to be a single nationwide list and that organ allocation should proceed without regard to which OPO actually procured the organs. (The logistical hurdles, not matters of right or principle, led to this plan's demise.) The critical point is not whether government action will actually impose such a single-list policy; the critical point is the undoubted right of the government, under the present system, to take such action. Public policy makers may not choose to set the nation's rules for organ allocation directly, but they can do so. Ten years ago, they could not refuse to certify an OPO that lacked an associated transplant hospital, nor could they intervene in practices involving the export of organs overseas.

Conclusion

The terms of the debate on organ sharing have undergone a fundamental revision in a very short time. Indeed, until 1986, there was no debate. Human organs for transplant belonged to the surgeons who excised them. Their use was in the surgeons' hands, and decisions regarding who received a transplant were dependent on the surgeons' understanding of their ethical responsibilities to their patients and their technical views on clinical matters. What consistency there was in organ distribution, and what justice and equity there were, derived from the similarities of training and values to be found among transplant surgeons. There was no other accountability.

Today there is lively and sometimes acrimonious debate over all aspects of organ sharing. The locus of the debate is not the local OPO or hospital but national organizations. The participants include not only medical professionals but also federal bureaucrats, congressional members and staffs, patient groups, academic immunologists, social scientists, and ethicists. The issues have broadened even more strikingly than the participants. Where once the critical issue was clinical efficacy, now considerations of costs, data quality, social equity, health policy, competition, and power over Medicare are all hotly contested and of immediate consequence.

These unprecedented changes reflect the convergence of developments inside and outside the transplant community. The central forces driving the changes are growth and technological development, and they are connected. In two decades, the transplant system has tripled in size. The number of organs transplanted has tripled, new kinds of transplants have become possible, the number of transplant centers has increased dramatically, and the number of people awaiting transplants has also grown commensurately. It is estimated that over thirty-five thousand Americans are currently living with another person's organ in their body. New drugs and techniques have made heart and liver transplantation possible and kidney transplantation far more effective. The magnitude of these developments has concentrated public, media, and political attention on the organ procurement and transplantation system.

New medical technology makes good press, especially when it affects the lives of children or when it can involve the heart, a muscle connected with much cultural symbolism. The media became fascinated, and so did the public. Appeals for donors on TV talk shows and appeals by the president did not go unheeded. Nor did tearful requests by the families of children in need.

The media coverage alone might have been enough to lure politicians into the fray, but other factors also beckoned. The costs of transplantation were becoming an issue, not only as a direct expense but also as a symbol of high-technology medicine and as an example of the need to ration medical care. The technology of nonrenal transplantation raised questions of new coverage and new programs.

In contrast to the stable pre-1984 period, significant segments of the transplant community were ready to invite political involvement. The fastest-growing and most visible portion of the community, nonrenal transplantation, was turning to the government, and indeed to the public and the media, for support, legitimation, and resources. Within the kidney transplantation community, physicians favoring organ sharing on the basis of tissue matching looked for support to overcome their disadvantages vis-à-vis those who would not share organs on this basis. There were also professional conflicts between immunologists and the more clinically oriented surgeons, as well as the growing desire of transplant coordinators to carve an area of autonomy for themselves. (Their ability to make this desire significant was itself a function of the increased size and cost of the organ procurement system that they operated.)

These various forces could not dominate the transplant community, and only the nonrenal surgeons could even be considered major powers in it. However, they could split the community, give the public more than one voice to hear from, and—most important—make vigorous resistance to outside involvement difficult. So while the transplant community as a whole did not welcome government involvement, it could not consistently oppose it. It repeatedly found itself forced to choose the lesser of two evils, the less interventionist of two proposals, and attempt to co-opt what it could not prevent. Of course, there were always the benefits of federal funding to consider.

The National Task Force on Organ Transplantation was not greeted with enthusiasm, but it seemed harmless enough, and it was to make a recommendation regarding federal payment for immunosuppressive drugs. A transplant surgeon became the chairwoman. Payment for the drugs was recommended, but so was the formation of a national organ-sharing network. The network might not really be needed, in the community's view, but there was a considerable amount of money associated with it, and the government might go ahead without them. So UNOS applied for the contract while resisting altering its character as an association of transplant surgeons, but the pressure and the opportunity could not be resisted, and it compromised. There would be public accountability if not public control.

So step by step, organ distribution was chivied and seduced into the public arena, with the transplant community never quite understanding the price that accompanied the added resources and power. Now UNOS finds itself defending a conception and a system that most of its members and virtually all of its leadership would have rejected with indignation a handful of years ago. The reality of UNOS continues to be professional dominance, but the exercise of that dominance is now both somewhat limited and far more accountable. Surgeons continue to dominate all aspects of decision making, but they do not have a monopoly on the positions of power in UNOS, and they find themselves accountable to others for the decisions they make. For example, while UNOS decided to ignore Congress's views on foreign nationals, it nevertheless published its policies in a formal manner, distributed them widely (through the *Federal Register*), and responded to public criticisms with public answers. This is a far cry from a major urban hospital quietly deciding that a Saudi princess ought to get the next kidney. In the same way, the organization's handling

151

of a complaint against one of its member OPOs illustrates this mix of continuity in policy but acceptance of public review. A hospital-based OPO was accused in the local media of giving unfair preference to the patients of its medical director over the patients of doctors affiliated with a nearby hospital. UNOS sent a team to examine the charges. If true, these charges would have required the expulsion of the OPO. The team deemed the specific charges of inequity unfounded but revealed that the OPO's sharing criteria were insufficiently documented and its record keeping of allocation decisions was incomplete. The OPO agreed to make the necessary changes.

One view holds that UNOS has changed nothing: the OPO wasn't penalized, nor was it required to change its policies. UNOS, one might say, deferred to local power and rallied behind a coprofessional. However, a local OPO was called to account for its practices by a national organization and as a result of public outcry. In the end, it was required to expose its behavior to public scrutiny. Whether this is viewed as the minimalist response of a conservative organization or the tentative intervention of a new organization feeling its way, it was an intervention by national forces in a local matter in a manner totally inconceivable five years earlier. What is more, it was intervention by an organization led by the mainstream leadership of the transplantation community.

It is doubtful that the transplantation community realizes the extent of the changes that have occurred. Partly, the realization is clouded by the fact that the community is involved in a determined defense of UNOS against forces seeking further to "socialize" organ distribution. HHS's attempts to claim direct government oversight of all organ-sharing policies were resisted by the transplant surgeons on new grounds. Several years ago, surgeons would have stood on medical ethics, medical expertise, and the defense of patients. Now they attempt to rally patients, families, related organizations, associations, and advocacy groups. Rather than claim that HCFA goals are unacceptable because they interfere with the practice of medicine, they now claim that there is already extensive "government surveillance," "government authority," and "public accountability," and they cite as precedents professional review organizations such as the Joint Commission on Hospital Accreditation and the National Association of Securities Dealers!

In recent years, the nation and the transplant community have accepted a new answer to the question "Whose organs are these?" The organs, it has been decided, are public property, and the organ distribution system is the public's trustee for them. The granting of public resources and public power and the insistence that those resources and that power be exercised under public oversight are expressions of the same phenomenon, the movement of organ distribution into the public domain. Coincident with the broadening of the people involved has been the broadening of the terms of debate. Who ought to have an opportunity to receive a transplant is a question that can no longer be answered with the smug answers of years ago. If the question had even been put a few years ago, the answer would simply have been that whoever is best suited is offered an organ. Now different views vie for a role in defining who is "best suited." Alternative allocation systems are now defended in public debate, and equity as well as efficiency must be considered and defined. Physicians dominate the debate, through knowledge as well as power, but they must justify their actions now as trustees of the public. The organs are no longer theirs.

6

Transplantation
and Public Policy

A SURGICAL OPERATION is a paid performance, complete with stage, actors, and props. Attention is naturally centered on the main attraction—the beauty and functionality of the operating suite, the heart-lung machine, the virtuoso performance of the surgeons. Little thought is given to any of the many other aspects of the process that brings all these necessary ingredients together. This is as it should be. This process is important, but only as all pieces of a whole are important. It does not contain any unique elements or any challenges of a qualitatively distinct kind, just the ordinary, if difficult, logistical demands facing any producer. Evaluation is therefore legitimately of a unitary event—is the surgery a success?

A transplant operation is different. The procurement of a human organ is qualitatively distinct from the acquisition of a piece of advanced medical hardware. In the first instance, it cannot be purchased. It can be obtained only by the conjoining of a person's death and a family's altruism. In our society— indeed, in all human societies—a dead body is a sacred object. It demands respect and must be treated accordingly. These considerations do not apply to other medical activities where all the necessary components are commodities purchased at market prices. The central question for public policy is whether the differences between transplantation and other high-technology

155

medicine requires that transplants be treated differently from a public perspective and, if so, what those differences ought to be.

From one perspective, organ transplantation is archetypical of American medicine during the second half of the twentieth century. It is costly and is meant to respond to a catastrophic health failure. It is essential to the well-being of transplant recipients, but their number is small. Like many forms of high-technology medicine, transplantation is a dramatic medical intervention that prolongs life at the cost of imposing a permanent dependence on continued medical treatment. It saves lives and increases chronic illness.

Its social and political configuration also have much in common with other expensive medical technologies. The procedures involved are esoteric, inaccessible even to 90 percent of physicians, but the professionals and institutions involved are wholly committed to it on philosophical grounds, and they benefit from it materially. They, and their patients, represent a compact, self-aware, and vehement lobby. Finally, like most other high-technology medical procedures, transplantation is dependent on public policy and public money. Government probably pays for two-thirds of all organ transplants directly; government regulations and funding make the entire infrastructure of organ procurement and distribution possible.

For these reasons, one could discuss transplantation, bypass surgery, chemotherapy for cancers, magnetic resonance imaging, lithotripsy, and a host of other medical innovations in like terms. All raise similar questions of rationing, priorities, and the connection between public resources and personal health. Indeed, many people frame consideration of transplantation in just this way and focus on transplantation, because of its visibility, drama, and cost, as an emblem of all that is bad (or good) about high-technology medicine.

But concentration on similarities can obscure differences. Organ transplantation is unique in its dependence on a "medical device" that cannot be manufactured or replicated, whose supply is beyond the ken of the medical system and largely outside the boundaries of the market system. Even as commodities, organs differ in that their shortage cannot be compensated for in any direct way by an increase in other investment. When rationing is discussed in transplantation, it refers to the allocation of organs; in all other contexts, it is about the allocation of money. Throughout the Western world, the buying and selling of organs are prohibited. All organs are obtained as gifts, and by laws strongly consistent with public preferences, these are free and voluntary donations, altruistically motivated. Public policy must therefore reflect the unique status of transplantation as an area of high-tech medicine unlike any other. Only in transplantation is fostering altruism a necessary part of public policy.

Transplantation as Technology

The transplantation of a human organ is a complex and demanding surgical procedure. Liver transplants in particular make extraordinary demands on surgical teams. But the true character of transplantation as advanced medical technology is best understood in a wider framework. Recipient selection and preparation are an equally critical part of a successful transplantation program. This involves the clinical evaluation of the recipient and, in the case of renal transplantation, skilled work in HLA typing.

157

Long-term success is also highly dependent on the management of the rejection reaction, a process that requires maintaining a delicate balance between tissue rejection and immunosuppression.

Advances in immunosuppressive agents have made long-term success more likely and the process of obtaining it more complex because several chemical agents are now available that differ in terms of efficacy and side effects. Organ transplantation therefore requires teams of medical specialists, large investments of hospital time, and the long-term management of some of the most advanced and most powerful pharmaceuticals in existence. The only classic element of high technology it lacks is dependence on large and expensive machinery. In its dependence on biotechnology rather than machine technology, it may not fall short of the classic model so much as presage the development of medical technology during the next decades.

Reservations about high-technology medicine can easily be applied to organ transplantation. Liver and heart transplantation save lives, and heart-lung and lung transplants have the potential for doing so. Renal transplantation improves the quality of life for its patients. In this sense, transplantation is a successful clinical approach. But the number of people who can benefit from a transplant is small, and the lifesaving nature of this approach reflects the fact that it is initiated at the end of a disease process. The entire transplantation system, therefore, serves to save the lives of relatively few extremely ill patients who will be dependent on medical care for the rest of their now extended lives.

Transplantation is expensive, even though the organ is donated as a gift. The direct cost of a kidney transplant is a rather "modest" $35,000, whereas a liver transplant may cost $500,000. The real cost of these procedures is much higher still, when procurement and aftercare are factored in. The direct cost of immunosuppressive drugs can easily reach $7,000 per year, and even without rejection episodes, frequent consultation with and evaluation by medical teams are necessary. These two aspects of transplantation—that it benefits relatively few people and requires lifetime aftercare—are the source of reservations about public support for this and other high-technology medicine. Many transplant recipients cannot reenter the work force, and all face high future medical costs and uncertain future health statuses. All of this imposes a heavy financial burden on society via direct payment for treatment, insurance premiums for health care, and income support programs.

To these substantive concerns might be added a kind of process concern. We know the present but not the future. Changes in transplantation procedures are largely beyond the control of policy makers and the public, so present decisions may commit us to unknown and uncontrollable futures. Technically, transplantation is evolving constantly. New procedures are under development, and some may have important implications for costs and volume. New immunosuppressive drugs are now coming on the market whose use may become mandatory as "best practice," and their cost may be high. New techniques are being developed that may alter both the demand and the supply of organs. Pancreas transplants are still experimental but, if successful, may become common. Recent experimentation with partial liver transplantation might lead to an explosion in the supply of transplantable livers.

Medical technologies build their own constituencies, whose

calls for supportive policies are likely to grow more powerful over time. The constituencies for transplantation are typical. At their center are the doctors and scientists who have a professional commitment to transplantation—transplant surgeons, immunologists, histocompatibility experts, and others. These professionals advance scientific and clinical arguments about the effectiveness and appropriateness of organ transplantation. In addition, they often play a role in mobilizing the patients who represent the other strand of transplant's political constituency. In this context, the small scale and dramatic nature of organ transplantation is an advantage. Identifiable human beings will benefit from public support for transplantation—or die if that support is not forthcoming. In public forums, on TV talk shows, and at congressional committee meetings, it is hard to criticize a treatment for saving so few when three of the people it could save are sitting in the room with you.

As the range of procedures expands and as new approaches are developed, these constituencies grow. Once the first steps in public support are taken, refusing the second and third steps becomes more difficult to defend. If the government will pay for immunosuppressive drugs for kidney recipients, why refuse such payment to heart recipients now or liver or pancreas recipients in the future?

Rationing Medical Care

Such concerns have forced policy makers to seek rationales for evaluating medical technologies of many kinds, including transplantation. In several instances, this has led to a decision to treat transplantation like all other high-technology medicine and to refuse to use public funds to pay for it. State Medicaid programs have been in the forefront of this approach, some deciding that Medicaid would not cover transplantation. Some of these states have parsimonious Medicaid programs, and their exclusion of transplantation services is consistent with overall limits on coverage. Oregon, however, has a generous program, yet an explicit decision was made to exclude transplantation on rationing grounds. The state legislature decided that its limited Medicaid resources ought to be concentrated to provide "basic" medical care services (although Oregon could not ultimately proceed with its rationing plan).

Underlying all such limitations on the coverage of certain procedures is the idea that while everyone may be entitled to some basic package of medical services, this package does not include every possible treatment. What that package ought to consist of and the criteria for inclusion are still matters of debate, but the central tests are widely agreed on. These tests are cost-benefit-oriented and have two connected aspects. The more general involves how medical care money can best be used to protect the health of the entire population, and the more specific addresses how it can best be used on an individual basis.

The Oregon legislature had decided that money spent on prenatal care produced more health benefits per dollar than money spent on transplantation, so the former should be part of the package and not the latter. This is hardly a disputable contention and provides an overarching rationale for preferring primary care to tertiary care and, for that matter, for preferring the care of the young over that of the old.

At a more micro level, the same principle can be applied to individual treatments. Each medical treatment can be evaluated in terms of the likelihood of its success and the amount and quality of additional life it ensures versus its cost. This approach concentrates on cost and benefits on an individual level. Very few policy makers and no public payers of health care are prepared to apply the broadest criteria in a systematic fashion. To do so would enforce a radical restructuring of American health care, and a good deal of tertiary medicine and geriatric medicine would not survive. Instead, the application of cost-benefit criteria is generally made at the margin by applying it to new technologies as they arise.

A decision to exclude transplantation from coverage by any payment program can be attacked on these narrow grounds. It can be asked whether the system will pay for treatment that is less cost-effective than transplantation solely because it has done so in the past. The standard question (because the most unanswerable) concerns the willingness of Medicaid (or a private insurer) to pay for the treatment of pancreatic cancer, which is almost wholly ineffectual and can be very expensive. In this case, an ordering of treatments by cost-benefit analysis would place transplantation above many procedures already covered by both public and private insurers, and transplantation ought to be given its fair place in the queue of treatments ranked strictly by cost-benefit criteria. If the Medicaid system has sufficient money to cover equally effective procedures, it ought to be included. If not, it ought to be excluded.

This reasoning assumes that organ transplantation is morally indistinguishable from other medical procedures. It holds that all aspects of medical policy-making are subject to a cost-benefit analysis where economics defines the cost and medicine the benefits. But some key parts of the organ transplantation process are outside both the economic and the medical systems. The decision to refuse public funding for any organ transplant high-lights the basic issue of whether public policy regarding trans-plantation must be different from policy in other areas. As a rationing decision of Medicaid dollars, it is a defensible action. A more complex issue is the adequacy of the policy in terms of its impact on the rationing of human organs.

Commodity Rationing

Organ transplantation is limited by the supply of organs, not by the money health insurers are willing to pay. The demand for transplants exceeds the supply to such a degree that a deci-sion by a payer not to cover transplantation has *only* distribu-tional impacts. When a state Medicaid office refuses to pay for a liver transplant, the number of liver transplants is not de-creased, the total amount of money spent on liver transplants is not decreased, and the demand for liver transplants is not decreased in any meaningful way. All that happens is that a Medicaid recipient doesn't receive the organ and someone else does.

No expenditure of money can directly increase the supply of transplantable organs. The law does not allow the price of organs to rise, the usual response of the market to an excess of demand over supply. There are very few current analogies for this state of affairs. Historically, the situation is more com-mon. Wartime rationing is the most obvious example. Under those circumstances, the demand for gasoline, for example, may be far greater than the supply, but a social and political deci-sion is made not to let the price of fuel rise high enough to drive most people out of the market. People must be able to get to work, shop, and get around, so it is important that a commodity in short supply not be frittered away on luxury consumption. Rationing decisions can also be based on equity: butter is rationed so that everyone may have some. Rationing also shows the population that everyone is being asked to share the burden of sacrifice equally. Several of those considerations support a decision to ration human organs outside the market system.

The Implications of Altruism

The most difficult decision to understand and defend in our age is a moral one. If a man kills an elderly clerk while robbing a store, we have a clear sense of his motivation. Only if we discover that he did it for reasons other than money are we surprised or taken aback. If he killed for fun or excitement, we consider him insane; not so if he killed for money. Aberrations from economic motivation require explanation, and the explanations are generally received with skepticism. But organ transplantation is rooted in noneconomic realities, and these are reflected in policy.

The foundation of transplantation policy is that the dead are somehow sacred, but at the same time, their organs are valuable commodities. In one sense, their bodies are regarded as inviolate and cannot be used as a means to any end. In practice, of course, sacred objects are often defiled; medical students pull pranks with cadavers, and soldiers make barricades of them. But these transgressions reinforce the sacredness of the dead precisely because they are viewed as transgressions and engender guilt or hilarity. Every state in the nation (perhaps every nation in the world) has laws defining how the dead are to be treated and providing penalties for disrespectful treatment.

If this aura about the sacredness of bodies did not exist, organ transplantation policy would certainly be based on traditional economic principles. The dead would be bought and sold; they would probably be eaten. But if human bodies were *only* sacred, organ transplantation would be impossible because organs could never be removed from them. This is not farfetched: Orthodox Jewish practices make transplantation difficult in Israel, and traditional Chinese beliefs make it even rarer in Asia. What makes organ transplantation possible in the West are mechanisms that allow transmogrification of a sacred body into a utilitarian source of lifesaving materials. The key is to allow the organ to become a useful object without becoming an economic commodity.

As indicated in Chapter Three, families of donors justify their actions by reference to altruism. In their minds, no desecration is involved if their relative's body can be used on behalf of the well-being of a living stranger. The profit motive has been excluded from organ distribution. What has taken its place are considerations of equity.

Equity is not a primary concern of market systems but must be a concern of systems built on altruism. When people make a gift of their relative's body, they know it won't be sold to the highest bidder, but they also want to know that it will be used in the best possible way. The medical professionals involved also expect their uncompensated efforts to have ethically valid outcomes. These expectations are an accepted part of present policy. The obligations of the transplant system to families and medical professionals grow out of the fact that they have made an ethical investment in the transplantation system, and it in turn owes them practices on an equal moral plain. Equity is the moral coin of the transplantation system because it is primarily a distributional system.

The procurement system has an obligation to treat both the body and the relatives with care and respect, and the entire system has an implied obligation to use the gift effectively. But underlying all of this is a recognized obligation that the gift be distributed fairly, based on the need of the recipient.

The Implications of Equity

The implementation of fairness has already been discussed, but its policy implications are broader. By law and practice, all families must be given a chance to permit organ or tissue donation. Policy does not, however, let the donor designate the recipient, nor may the families even be told who received their gift. We know from survey data that the public accepts these terms and asks only that the organs be distributed on the basis of medical need. They give to help others and are satisfied when assured that that help will be distributed fairly.

The organ distribution and transplantation system is committed to fulfilling these expectations and has a number of reasons for doing so. The ethical arguments have been touched on—organs are donated out of the highest moral motivations, and the transplant system has an obligation to maintain equivalent standards or break faith with the givers. In addition to being morally unacceptable, acting in bad faith could endanger the supply of organs. A widespread fear among OPOs is that mistrust of the transplantation system could cause families to refuse to donate. This fear may be well founded. When a series of stories indicated that the University of Pittsburgh was allocating organs unfairly, donation rates dropped. Equally, mistrust on the part of doctors and nurses might lead to decreased referrals. From a purely instrumental point of view, a system based on voluntary donations must be above reproach. In this context, it must be seen as allocating organs according to fair, objective, and medically defensible criteria.

There are honest differences among professionals as to what the correct scientific criteria should be. For the system's reputation to remain solid, agreement on criteria isn't essential, only that the terms of the debate be acceptable. Discussion about recipient location, for example, is permissible; discussion over race or ability to pay is not.

The Policy Question

Nonrenal transplantation is not covered by Medicaid payment rules in every state. The federal government's Medicare program will pay for liver transplants only under rare and limited conditions. Most transplant hospitals will accept transplant candidates only if some payment source can be located beforehand. Uninsured and underinsured Americans are therefore effectively excluded from consideration.

Many people have questioned the wisdom of these restrictions, but the broader question concerns their legitimacy. The organ transplantation system is supported and directed by the federal government to a degree that is unique in American medicine. This reflects Congress's acceptance of the public nature of the system's responsibilities—the duty to deliver the "gift of life" to people in need without regard to extraneous social characteristics. Rich families and poor, of all ethnicities, are equally asked to give and equally denied the right to select the recipient. Medical suitability, logistical limitations, and time on the waiting

167

list are the only criteria the transplant system formally applies to allocation decisions. Since the mid 1980s, the federal government has taken the view that the public interest requires the systematic application of these standards of behavior.

In its 1986 report, the National Task Force on Organ Transplantation pointed out that increases in the costs of immunosuppressive drugs were undermining the practical application of this policy of equitable organ distribution. Congress acted immediately to alter the End-Stage Renal Disease program to cover the cost of these drugs. Because this could be done within the framework of the ESRD program, it could be seen as a technical adjustment to the coverage provided by that law.

Technical innovation in transplantation has hardly been limited to improved immunosuppressive drugs. When the ESRD program was initiated, only kidney transplantation was clinically feasible. Now over one-third of all organ transplants involve nonrenal organs. Hearts, livers, and other nonrenal organs are procured exactly as kidneys are. The same institutions approach the same families. The same obligations apply. Yet because renal and nonrenal transplants are paid for differently, organ allocation differs, and many Americans are financially barred from receiving a nonrenal transplant.

The issue is which responsibility should take primacy—the responsibility of the transplant system to deal equitably with all organs or the responsibility of the payment system to set priorities. Rationing of medical care is a reality. If all people are not to be entitled to all available care, policies must be developed to differentiate covered and uncovered care. If Medicaid officials decide that they will not pay for lithotripsy or Congress declines to cover outpatient drugs under Medicare, these are legitimate rationing decisions. They may not be wise or generous, but they do not conflict with other commitments. Analogous decisions not to pay for adult liver transplants or heart transplants for Medicaid recipients, however, do conflict with the commitment made to donor families. The organ procurement system does not let families select recipients and promises to do the selecting for them based on medical need, but other arms of government exclude patients who are unable to pay.

Consistency is the hobgoblin of little minds but the foundation of equitable public policy. Either reimbursement policies or organ procurement policies need to be changed. There are good reasons not to change transplant policy. Organs are in shorter supply than money, and altruism is a social value that is rare enough as it is. The financial cost of eliminating financial barriers to access to transplantation is low; the social cost of breaking faith with donor families is high.

The federal government has been resistant to developing entitlement programs for organ transplantation because of its experience with the ESRD program. But less than 10 percent of the cost of the ESRD program goes to renal transplantation. Individually, transplants are expensive, but total system costs are limited by the number of cadaveric donors, of whom there were only about 4,500 in 1992. Even the most optimistic estimates do not foresee an enormous increase in that number, so the total cost of organ transplantation simply cannot skyrocket. The costs to public payers for covering the relatively small percentage of individuals now excluded would be much smaller yet. Financially, the risks are negligible.

The social costs are also low. In pure cost-benefit terms,

169

providing funding to everyone who undergoes organ transplantation when we don't provide generalized funding for other, more widely needed services is not sensible. Arguments could be made that the money going to transplant procedures could go elsewhere, but these complaints are by no means unanswerable. Transplantation is different, and it has the strong support of the American public. Through required request laws, brain death laws, the OPTN contract, the National Organ Transplantation Act, and the ESRD program, the government has already singled transplantation out in many ways and accepted responsibility for it. Broadening entitlement to excluded groups is not a large or discontinuous step but rather a natural progression of current policy.

Since current policy is *federal* policy, the burden of expanding transplant funding ought to sit with Congress. Congressional policy has declared human organs a national resource, and federal money already pays for the bulk of organ transplantation. It would be a small step for changes in the Medicare and Medicaid laws to ensure that all Americans not otherwise insured would have any needed organ transplant covered by these programs. The decision to cover immunosuppressive drugs for kidney recipients was the only way to protect the goals of the ESRD program in an altered technical environment. The only way to protect the values and goals of our present organ transplantation system is to extend federal coverage to all organ transplantation.

Altruism and Public Policy

We expect people to act according to different values in different spheres of their lives. Within families and among friends,

170

we expect generosity and kindness. In interactions with the world at large, market exchange relationships prevail. The concept of community is squeezed between these spheres. Within a community, some of the values of family life are applied to strangers. One serves a community by donating time, efforts, talent, or money to the betterment of strangers. A woman serves on the board of a hospital, contributes to a family shelter, helps construct a playground. Her rewards include the respect of others, a sense of doing the right thing, and membership in an improved community. The beneficiaries are primarily people she doesn't know, and not just at the hospital, shelter, or playground. Community-spirited action gives birth to community by defining a set of strangers entitled to be treated with kindness and generosity. Those who neither build nor play on the swings benefit insofar as they now partake of a relationship that is more complex and more forgiving than that of the economic marketplace.

All valued human relationships contain elements of community, if only in an attenuated, even mythological way. Nations survive on this. We are encouraged to "buy American!" even though we know the workers in Flint no better than those in Osaka. We clamor to "free the American hostages" even though they are as much strangers to us as the Swiss hostages or the Lebanese captors. Yet because they are Americans, we accept a greater obligation for their welfare than for the welfare of others. This sense of community is the glue that holds us together.

The origins and underpinnings of community are complex, subtle, and not easily manipulated. Where they exist, they are often robust, and where they don't, they are generally intractably absent. Nevertheless, opportunities to foster community are not common and should not be squandered. Organ donation is such an opportunity; indeed, it is almost a unique opportunity. The circumstances are profoundly tragic, but they generate the emotions that tie people closer together.

The donation of organs is a community-building action of great emotional and symbolic potency. The gift is to a stranger; it binds the stranger to the givers in powerful ways. The stranger's gain mitigates the family's loss; a service is rendered in both directions, between people who will never meet. The givers assert their membership in a community in a tangible and symbolic way. Though the recipients benefit directly and critically from their membership in this community, all members benefit indirectly. Each of us knows that we could find ourselves in either the giver's or the receiver's role. Most of us state our willingness to engage in that "gift relationship" if the circumstances arise. It is a willingness to enter into a sacred relationship with people who must then be seen as more than simply strangers.

Of almost equal importance, an organ donation is a gift made possible by public action. The community, acting through public bodies, provides the mechanism to make this altruistic act meaningful. By supporting organ donation, the community demonstrates that it values altruism and the strengthening of bonds among its members. It further legitimizes the act of giving and the efforts of the people who make the gift possible and in doing so legitimizes itself as a valuable and real community of people. In our society, there are few opportunities to reinforce the bonds of empathy, mutual help, and even love that communities ultimately depend on. Altruism is valuable not merely for itself but also for the coherence it encourages.

Government tax policy encourages charity, and publicly supported volunteer programs encourage mutual help; President Bush spoke of becoming "a kinder and gentler" nation. Organ transplantation depends for its existence on the presence of these virtues. Public policy has institutionalized them in its approach to organ transplantation. It is important that no one be excluded from this vision of a community made possible by kindness to strangers.

References

Aiken-O'Neill, P. Letter from the Eye Bank Association of America. 1992.

Bergstrom, C., and Gabel, H. "Organ Donation and Organ Retrieval Program in Sweden, 1990." *Journal of Transplant Coordination,* 1991, *1,* 47–50.

Caplan, A., and Welvang, P. "Are Required Request Laws Working? Altruism and the Procurement of Organs and Tissues." *Clinical Transplantation,* 1989, *3,* 170–176.

Cleveland, S. "Changes in Human Tissue Donor Attitudes, 1969–1974." *Psychosomatic Medicine,* 1975, *37,* 306–312.

Cook, D., and Terasaki, P. "Impact of HLA Matching and Pretransplant Transfusion on Transplant Outcome." *Transplantation Proceedings,* 1988, *20,* 224–248.

Eggers, P. "Trends in Medical Reimbursement for End-State Renal Disease, 1974–1979." *Health Care Financing Administration Review,* Fall 1984, pp. 31–38.

Eggers, P. "Effects of Transplantation on the Medicare End-State Renal Disease Program." *New England Journal of Medicine,* 1988, *318,* 223–229.

Evans, R., Orrans, C., and Uscher, W. "The Potential Supply of Organ Donors." *JAMA,* 1992, *267,* 239–246.

Evans, R., and others. *National Heart Transplantation Study.* Report to the Health Care Financing Administration, 1984.

Eye Bank Association of America. *Newsletter,* Mar. 26, 1992.

Fox, R., and Swazey, J. "The Democratization Dialysis Law: 92–603." In Fox, R., and Swazey, J. *The Courage to Fail.* Chicago: University of Chicago Press, 1973.

Gallup Organization. *Attitudes and Opinions of the American Public Toward Kidney Donation.* Princeton, N.J.: Gallup Organization, 1983.

Gallup Organization. *Attitudes and Opinions of the American Public Toward Kidney Donation.* Princeton, N.J.: Gallup Organization, 1985.

General Accounting Office. *Organ Transplants.* Washington, D.C.: General Accounting Office, 1992.

"HCFA Releases 1991 End-Stage Renal Disease Program Data." *Nephrology News and Issues,* Feb. 1993, p. 12.

Health Care Financing Administration. *Program Highlights, 1991.* Washington, D.C.: Health Care Financing Administration, 1992.

Intergovernmental Health Policy Project. *Review of States' Brain Death, Organ Donor, and Procurement Legislation.* Report to the Health Research and Services Administration, 1985.

Lowy, C. "Tissue Groups and Kidney Sharing: Sociocultural Aspects of a Medical Controversy." *Journal of Technology Assessment in Health Care,* forthcoming.

Manninen, D., and Evans, R. "Public Attitudes and Behavior Regarding Organ Donation." *JAMA,* 1985, *253.*

Moore, B., Clarse, G., Lewis, B. R., and Malhet, N. P. "Public Attitudes Toward Kidney Transplantation." *British Medical Journal,* 1976, *1,* 629–631.

Nathan, H., and others. "Estimation and Characterization of the Potential Organ Donor Pool in Pennsylvania." Unpublished paper, 1991.

National Kidney Foundation. "Public Attitudes on Organ Donation." *UNOS Update,* Feb. 1992.

National Task Force on Organ Transplantation. *Report on Immunosuppressive Therapies.* Report to the U.S. Department of Health and Human Services, 1985.

National Task Force on Organ Transplantation. *Organ Transplantation.* Report to the U.S. Department of Health and Human Services, 1986.

"New HCFA Rules May Squash Kidneys for Foreigners." *Nephrology News and Issues,* Mar. 1987, p. 12.

Opelz, G. "The Benefit of Exchanging Donor Kidneys Among Transplant Centers." *New England Journal of Medicine,* 1988, *318,* 1289–1297.

Opelz, G. "Analysis of Risk Factors in Renal Transplantation." Paper presented to the New England Organ Bank, Boston, 1991.

Prottas, J. *Organizational Effects in Organ Procurement.* Report to the Health Care Financing Administration, 1982.

Prottas, J. "Obtaining Replacements: The Organizational Framework of Organ Procurement." *Journal of Health Politics, Policy, and Law,* 1983, 8, 235–250.

Prottas, J. *Analysis and Evaluation of the U.S. Organ Procurement System: Hospital and Independent Agencies Compared.* Report to the Health Care Financing Administration, 1984.

Prottas, J. "The Structure and Effectiveness of the U.S. Organ Procurement System." *Inquiry,* 1985, *22,* 365–376.

Prottas, J. *The Organ Procurement and Distribution System in the United States.* Report to the Health Care Financing Administration, 1987.

Prottas, J. "Shifting Responsibilities in Organ Procurement: A Plan for Routine Referral." *JAMA,* 1988, *260,* 832.

Prottas, J. "The Organization of American Organ Procurement." *Journal of Health Politics, Policy, and Law,* 1989, *14,* 41–55.

Prottas, J., and Batten, H. *Attitudes and Incentives in Organ Procurement: Professional Attitudes.* Report to the Health Care Financing Administration, 1986a.

Prottas, J., and Batten, H. *The Attitudes of the American Public.* Report to the Health Care Financing Administration, 1986b.

Prottas, J., and Batten, H. "Health Professionals and Hospital Administrators in Organ Procurement: Attitudes, Reservations, and Resolutions." *American Journal of Public Health,* 1988, *78,* 643–645.

Prottas, J., and Batten, H. *Medical Professionals in New Jersey: Attitudes Toward Organ Procurement: A Comparison of National and New Jersey Attitudes.* Report to the New Jersey Department of Health, 1990.

Prottas, J., and Batten, H. *Causes of Failure to Transplant Cadaveric*

Human Organs. Report to the Health Care Financing Administration, 1991a.

Prottas, J., and Batten, H. "The Willingness to Give: The Public and the Supply of Transplantable Organs." *Journal of Health Politics, Policy, and Law,* 1991b, *16*, 121–134.

Prottas, J., Hecht, S., and Batten, H. *Changes in the Nation's Organ Procurement System, 1982–1986.* Report to the Health Care Financing Administration, 1987.

Salvatierra, C. "Optimal Use of Organs for Transplantation." *New England Journal of Medicine,* 1988, *318,* 1329–1331.

Schneider, A., and Flaherty, M. "The Challenge of a Miracle: Selling the Gift." *Pittsburgh Press,* Nov. 3, 1985, p. A18.

Stiller, C. *Organ Donation in the Eighties.* Ontario Ministry of Health, 1984.

United Network for Organ Sharing. *Update,* Sept. 1988.

United Network for Organ Sharing. *Update,* Feb.-Mar. 1989a.

United Network for Organ Sharing. *Update,* Oct. 1989b.

United Network for Organ Sharing. "Facts about Transplantation in the United States." *Update,* 1991a.

United Network for Organ Sharing. *Update,* Dec. 1991b.

United Network for Organ Sharing. *Update,* Oct. 1992.

Index

A

African-Americans: attitudes of, 54, 59–61, 64, 66–67, 71; as donors, 34–35
AIDS, and procurement, 27
Aiken-O'Neill, P., 51
Altruism: and public policy, 157, 164–166, 170–173; and public role, 49–50, 63–64, 65, 76
Animal organs, 5–6
Assisted voluntarism, 50
Austria, procurement in, 13, 32

B

Battelle Institute, and attitude survey, 62
Batten, H., 9–10, 31, 52, 56n, 57n, 59, 60n, 61, 62, 65n. 73n, 83, 84n, 86n, 89n, 92n, 94, 95, 100n, 101n
Benelux nations, procurement in, 32
Bergstrom, C., 54
Bone donors, number of, 4–5
Brain death: criteria for, 9, 14; and medical professionals, 80, 88–90, 99, 103–104
Brandeis University, and attitude survey, 62
Bush, G., 173
Bush administration, and distribution system, 48, 126, 136

C

Canada: attitudes in, 54; procurement in, 25
Caplan, A., 15, 50
Catastrophic Care Act of 1988, 132
Catholic church, and organ donations, 10
China, beliefs in, 165
Clarse, G., 54
Cleveland, S., 54
Cold ischemic time: and distribution issues, 119, 120–121, 123, 124; and logistics, 29
Community spirit, and public policy, 171–172
Conference of Commissioners on Uniform State Laws, 12
Cook, D., 121
Cornea donation, presumed consent for, 14, 51
Corneal transplants: and Jewish law, 10; number of, 4
Cross-matching: and distribution, 118–119, 120–125, 131; in procurement process, 30
Cyclosporine: and distribution system, 122, 131–132, 133–134; use of, 6. See also Immunosuppressive drugs

D

Death, declaration of, 27–28

179

U

Uniform Anatomical Gift Act (UAGA), 12–14, 28, 116
United Kingdom: attitudes in, 54; distribution in, 140; procurement in, 32, 38
United Network for Organ Sharing (UNOS), 2, 10, 35n, 39, 42, 126, 127, 142; and distribution system, 118–119, 137, 138–139, 141, 144–147, 151–152; in infrastructure, 17–18, 30
U.S. Department of Health and Human Services (HHS): and distribution system, 138, 143, 145–146, 147, 152–153; and procurement, 19, 44–45, 46, 47–48
Uscher, W., 42

V

Vascularized organ transplants, number of, 2
Voluntarism, assisted and passive forms of, 50–51

W

Warm ischemic time, 28
Wastage rate, acceptable, 47
Waxman, H., 135
Welvang, P., 15, 50

X

Xenografts, 5–6

There are more than fifteen thousand human organ transplants performed annually in the United States, and each year demand increases, outstripping the medical industry's ability to supply organs. Faced with this relative scarcity, policy makers and health care professionals are forced to question the basic policies of organ procurement. For example, should organ procurement continue to rely on voluntary donations? And are there organizational and policy solutions that could alleviate the continuing shortage of human organs?

The Most Useful Gift, written for health care managers and policy makers, is the first comprehensive guide to understanding the challenges human organ procurement professionals face. In it, Jeffrey Prottas explains the organizational, technological, and social dynamics that make organ transplantation possible, and he offers specific suggestions on how to improve organ procurement and deal with the natural shortage of available human organs.

By tracing the progress of the field from its beginning, Prottas shows how organ procurement organizations (OPOs) have improved the delivery and efficiency of transplantation to the point where the average OPO today is